# The
# Determined
# Patient

## How to Be a
## **Powerful Self-Advocate**
## and Take Charge of Your Health

**ROBERT DANZIGER, MD, MBA**
**AND**
**MARGARET GELLENS, MD**
*with Nancy Peske*

Published in the United States by Kamoh Publishing, Chicago, IL
For more information, please visit www.KamohInc.com

ISBN: 978-0-578-34127-9 (paperback)
ISBN: 978-0-578-34126-2 (eBook)

Cover design by Damonza

Printed in the United States of America

# CONTENTS

# INTRODUCTION

When confronted with a medical illness, whether your own or that of a loved one or friend, it's easy to feel lost and confused as you begin to navigate your way through the medical system with all its complexities. You want to get the care and treatment that's best for you—customized medicine is the future of medicine, after all. But that means you, as the patient, need to know how to do the kind of research that your physician may not be able to do for you for whatever reason. It's your health, and you can become an effective partner to your physician so that you get an accurate diagnosis or diagnoses and your treatment can be tailored to produce optimal results.

That's where *The Determined Patient* comes in.

A powerfully effective approach to researching all the best options for immediate and future treatment might make all the difference in your achieving optimal care and the best possible health outcome. That's especially true if you have a medical mystery and aren't willing to accept your current state of health—or you're faced with a disease or condition for which the prognosis is dire and you aren't sure what treatment is right for you as a unique individual.

It's increasingly common for patients today to have to change doctors often, making consistency of care a challenging goal. By becoming a determined patient, you can make up for gaps created by the difficulties physicians face in managing the cases of hundreds of patients who have ever-changing conditions and needs.

You'll also want to know how to achieve access to the highest quality health care, make the best decisions about what to do for your health, and follow through on those decisions. *The Determined Patient* will show you how to be a strong self-advocate who is confident, prepared, and effective as you partner with medical professionals in caring for your health, leaving no stone unturned as you seek the answers you deserve.

## Why We Wrote This Book

We are two physicians with over sixty years of combined experience in the world of medicine. Robert S. Danziger, MD, a cardiologist, has been an academic university professor, actively teaching, practicing medicine, and running an NIH-funded basic science laboratory studying heart failure and hypertension. Mary E. Gellens, MD, is a nephrologist (a kidney specialist) who has been a practicing physician, academic faculty member, and senior director in the medical device/pharmaceutical industry. We have seen that patients who partner with us experience better health outcomes—and we want that for every patient. Our work with seriously ill patients has convinced us there is a strong need for a tool to help them feel emboldened to take charge of their health care, and we want patients to be able to do the following:

- research their condition and develop expertise on it
- recognize the signs that they may have been misdiagnosed or have an undiagnosed condition on top of their primary one
- identify the best, most up-to-date specialists with whom to partner

- discover the latest information on treatments and perhaps even connect with key opinion leaders/researchers who can provide cutting-edge insights

- dialogue with their doctors effectively, even during short visits

- ask all the crucial questions

- feel entitled to answers that satisfy their need for information and guidance

- be honest with themselves and their medical team about any obstacles that are preventing them from following their doctor's orders

- research costs for procedures, tests, and medical care and even perhaps prevent large bills

- discover ongoing clinical trials they might participate in or benefit from in some other way, such as through a "compassionate care" program

- work with their primary physician in charting the best course forward in care, whether it involves different physicians, medical centers, treatments, and/or clinical trials

- discover and understand the latest research that can help them in making treatment decisions and understanding their condition

However, accomplishing all this is virtually impossible without understanding how to navigate the medical system, including how to switch physicians, find the best place for your care, and get new and experimental treatments when faced with the most difficult-to-treat diseases or medical conditions. This may include learning about research that is being done and working with a caregiver and/or advocate who will serve on a strong team you'll build to support you in your quest for optimal health.

When you have finished reading this book, we hope you will keep it on hand so you can turn to its resources again and again. Please note that *The Determined Patient* is not a substitute for medical care. However, it will empower you to partner effectively with the best possible medical professionals to work with you. You *can* optimize the care you receive and your health outcome—if you're willing to become a determined patient and powerful self-advocate.

## Chapter One

# BECOME A DETERMINED PATIENT

Kevin was under a lot of pressure with several tight deadlines at work, a son who was flunking out of school, and a wife who was unhappy. When he started experiencing frequent headaches that didn't respond to painkillers, he became concerned and scheduled an appointment with his family doctor. Kevin answered the usual questions about his medical history, received a general physical, and was told by his physician, "Your headaches seem to be stress related. Why don't you try aspirin and call me in a couple of weeks if you don't see any improvement?"

Deciding that stress was probably at the heart of his problem, Kevin started taking aspirin whenever he felt pain near his temples. However, the headaches continued. He scheduled another appointment with his doctor, who now advised him to take up yoga and meditation. These practices are known to relieve stress, so it wasn't bad advice for a man who was experiencing a tough time emotionally. But even after Kevin began going to a health club and doing exercise including yoga, he continued having headaches. At this point, he decided to take charge and do some research on his own.

Using the online site WebMD and the process of elimination, he discovered he had all the symptoms of giant cell arteritis, a condition involving inflammation of cells in the brain near the temples. Kevin discussed with his doctor what he had learned and had his self-diagnosis confirmed. He was prescribed the recommended treatment: a course of steroids. To Kevin's great relief, the headaches disappeared within a week. He was able to avoid the potential complications of giant cell arteritis, which can affect many arteries, potentially causing symptoms beyond just headaches..

While reading Kevin's story, were you thinking he was a hypochondriac and his doctor wasn't taking him seriously enough? Would you simply have trusted that your doctor knew best, or would you have done your own research? If your doctor's recommended treatment didn't work, how long would it have taken for you look further into whether you had the right diagnosis and treatment?

We hear stories like Kevin's all the time. The truth is that doctors who do thorough exams may miss things, and during a typical visit from a patient with a complaint, a physician has probably allotted only fifteen to twenty minutes per appointment to make a diagnosis. A typical doctor is probably seeing twenty-five to thirty patients a day and is likely to be caring for as many as a thousand patients. Your doctor might not think to ask about a family history of certain diseases, and you might not be aware of your full history. Kevin's condition, giant cell arteritis, is often genetic, but it isn't as well known as diabetes or heart disease. Your physician may not remember at that particular visit that a certain combination of symptoms might be related to a relatively obscure condition—and if you have been under a lot of stress, your doctor may mistakenly believe that's the origin of your health problem.

A physician and patient working together are more likely to reach the right diagnosis than a harried doctor taking a medical history from a patient who isn't sure what to report or what to ask. Unfortunately, doctors' visits have become too much like speed dating. That's why you—as a patient, potential patient, caretaker, or advocate—need to have strategies for overcoming the limitations of the health-care system. You have to learn how to become a determined patient who receives the best care and achieves the best outcomes by doing effective research and partnering with your medical providers.

Far too often, people will simply trust their doctors and do a minimum of research into some of the terms their physician uses. They aren't aware that their doctor is dealing with dozens of other patients, some of them very ill, along with doing hospital rounds, dictating notes, keeping up on new medical research, attending conferences, and trying to have a life outside of work, too. To provide optimal care, the best doctors *want* patients who team with them and participate in active, productive dialogues about how best to improve their patient's state of health. They want patients who are compliant with their orders and who speak up when they find compliance challenging. *It doesn't matter how effective a medication or treatment is if you don't follow through with it.*

Effective partnering makes your doctor's job much more effective, which can mean that you get better health care and even better outcomes. For example, when taking a history and performing a physical examination, a doctor is going to ask questions to understand your symptoms. So before you get to your appointment, make sure that whenever you experience the symptom, *you pay attention to it and record it.*

---

### Observing and Recording Your Symptoms

- Pay attention to the details of the symptom. If you're experiencing pain, figure out how to best describe what the pain feels like (aching? shooting?), what brings it on, and what makes it go away. If you're having vision problems, describe exactly what happens.

- Notice whether your symptom is associated with other symptoms. Are your headaches accompanied by nausea? Are you experiencing fatigue as well as shortness of breath?

- Make a note in a health app, calendar, or journal of the time you experienced your symptom. Does your pain happen shortly after you eat? When you've been looking at a computer or mobile device screen for a while? Around the same time every day?

- Observe whether the qualities of the symptom change. Has a dull pain turned into a sharp one? Has a rash spread or changed in appearance?

You are the expert on your symptoms, so when you get to your doctor's office, you'll want to describe them as best you can so you can help your doctor arrive at the correct diagnosis. It takes a team effort between patient and physician to come up with the right diagnosis as fast as possible with the fewest and least invasive tests possible.

## Which Patient Are You?

The stories of two patients, Eric and Bill, demonstrate the power of a determined patient. Both Eric and Bill had been referred to Dr. Danziger because they had complained of shortness of breath, which can be a sign of heart problems. Both had been seen by many consulting physicians and had a pile of medical records. When he came to his appointment, Eric brought all his records—it made quite a stack. In glancing through the papers, Dr. Danziger saw results from many unnecessarily repeated tests that included cardiac catheterizations and lung scans, tests that are both expensive and potentially dangerous.

There seemed to be minimal communication among the physicians, and Eric had little idea of what was going on. He said that he'd been confused by what his doctors had told him and was hoping Dr. Danziger could help. Each successive physician seemed not to know which tests had already been done and what the results were and simply ordered new ones. In an age of electronic record-keeping, his physicians should have been able to access Eric's medical records, but for whatever reason, the communication broke down. Eric was so busy managing his health issues that he had just gone along with the recommendation to retest, trusting his doctors knew what they were doing.

Another patient, Bill, came to Dr. Danziger's office with a carefully organized set of his medical records stored as documents on his smartphone. He understood why each test had been done. No tests had been repeated and only a few key ones had been performed—even though he had been to the same number of doctors that Eric had been to. Bill knew what was going on with his condition and his treatment and saw his doctors as partners in his health care. He was assertive in asking questions that he had prepared before each visit to his doctor.

We want you to become a more knowledgeable and empowered medical consumer like Bill was—and make no mistake, even if you aren't paying a lot out of pocket for medical treatment, you're a consumer. You have some choices about the doctors you work with, the clinics and hospitals you go to, and the testing that's done. We want you to ask more questions and not be embarrassed in doing so. When you're not a medical expert and you're worried about your health, it's easy to become overwhelmed and simply trust that your doctor will take care of everything and won't make any mistakes. However, if you don't pay very close attention to what's going on with your health and treatment, you may not get the results you would get if you were more proactive. If you are more like Eric, don't worry. We will help you gain confidence in your ability to work effectively with your doctors to get the best medical care and outcome that you can.

What's more, you'll learn in this book that even if you have no medical background, you might be able to diagnose yourself based on your own observations and research. Of course, you'll want to confirm your self-diagnosis with a medical professional and work with a quality medical team to get the care you need, but you might be underestimating your ability to do good, quality research on what's going on in your body.

As a self-motivated and informed patient, you can also find the best treatments and access the same up-to-date information your doctor uses to decide on how best to help you return to your previous state of health. If you barely made it through high school biology and don't know the difference between an intern and an internist, don't worry. We can help you become a self-directed and knowledgeable patient who lets no obstacle stand in the way of getting optimal care.

If you were given a dire prognosis or you are not getting the answers and improvement you want, you don't have to take a "wait and see" approach or accept your current state of health. Your doctor might not be aware of other treatment options for you. We believe that even if you're shy, you have difficulty confronting those you see as authority figures (those experts in white coats), or you have minimal knowledge about your body and your health, you can become a determined patient. We'll teach you how to do high-quality research, ask excellent questions, better understand your condition and possible treatments, and follow your physician's orders. We want you to have a "can-do" attitude, not a mind-set of "better just hope for the best and try to do what the doctor says."

While there may be a few doctors who would be uncomfortable having a proactive, well-informed patient sitting in front of them in an examination room, questioning their diagnoses and suggestions for treatments, the physicians we know want to be health-care partners with their patients. They know this will increase the odds of achieving the best possible outcomes.

### *"Maybe I don't have the right diagnosis."*

### *—Linda's Story*

The story of Linda illustrates how being a knowledgeable, self-motivated patient can make all the difference in your treatment and outcome. Linda, eighty-one, had gone to her primary care provider, who was a nurse practitioner, because her legs and ankles had started to swell, making her shoes feel tight. The nurse practitioner told her that the most common cause of leg and ankle swelling (also known as pedal edema) is by far heart failure and in an older person, it is almost always the cause. She explained that in all likelihood, Linda's heart wasn't pumping as well as it had when she was younger, causing fluid to collect in her feet. An echocardiogram showed some mild reduction in the rate at which Linda's heart relaxed after contracting to send blood through her body. That led the nurse practitioner to diagnose diastolic heart failure and begin to treat Linda with diuretics, the most common treatment for that particular condition.

The diuretic usually solves the problem of pedal edema when someone has diastolic heart failure, but in Linda's case, it didn't help. Because the swelling did not improve, the nurse practitioner increased the dosage of the medication. Linda began urinating more frequently, which happens when a patient is on a diuretic, but five weeks after this change in her treatment, the edema still showed no improvement.

Now that her condition had persisted for two months, Linda became a truly determined patient and did some internet research. Because she knew that her primary symptom was pedal edema and she had no shortness of breath, making heart failure a little less likely, she decided to find out what other causes of pedal edema have been identified. She knew that WebMD was an easy-to-read website directed at laypeople, so she checked there first. Under "pedal edema," it listed ten potential causes, each of which she considered. These included allergic reactions (she had no allergies); obstruction of flow (she had no idea what this was); a critical illness (to her knowledge, she was not critically ill; she just had swollen feet!); liver disease (she had no symptoms of jaundice and was not a drinker); pregnancy (she was too old for that); head trauma (she had none); and a variety of medications (she was on none of them). The one thing on the list that caught her eye was "low albumin," so she asked her nurse practitioner to do a simple blood test to measure her level. As it turned out, the level was very low.

Then, Linda became a super-determined patient and looked up "causes of low albumin." She came across www.UpToDate.com—a website for physicians that anyone can subscribe to for a small fee. There she read about nephrotic syndrome, a condition in which the kidneys send too much protein into the urine rather than processing it as they are supposed to. Linda asked her nurse practitioner to refer her to a specialist, specifically, a nephrologist (a kidney doctor), so that she could check out this possibility.

When Dr. Gellens met Linda, she affirmed that the diagnosis could be correct and ordered a urine test to check for high levels of albumin in the urine. The test results were positive, so a kidney biopsy was done to determine the cause of the high urine albumin. The biopsy showed Linda had minimal change disease, which can cause nephrotic syndrome. She was treated with medications: steroids, angiotensin-converting enzyme (ACE) inhibitors, and diuretics. She also made dietary changes to help her condition. Her symptoms resolved over time.

Linda's example is just one of many that have convinced the two of us that any time your condition or symptoms aren't improving, you should see a specialist and do your research.

### *"I have nothing to lose at this point."*

### —*Marcus's Story*

Marcus is a physician turned patient. A sixty-five-year-old cardiologist in perfect health (or so it seemed), Marcus started having abdominal pain. He initially thought it was related to an abdominal hernia, which was then repaired. However, the pain persisted, and he went to an internist, who ordered several tests and diagnosed pancreatic cancer stage IV—the worst possible news for him. Pancreatic cancer is particularly deadly.

First, Marcus sought out the best oncologists locally. Then he compared their recommended courses of action and found a consensus: a three-drug "cocktail" was considered the best treatment. However, the treatment would increase his life expectancy by only a few months. He immediately set out to learn everything he could about the disease.

Marcus decided to check online to see whether there were clinical trials for new potential treatments that might be more effective. He found a clinical trial for a new approach to treating the cancer that involved something called microbubbles, which make it easier to get the chemotherapeutic agent to the cancerous cells. Marcus knew that if he actually participated in the trial, he would only have a 50 percent chance of receiving the new therapy: He could end up in the "control group" that would receive the established treatment or a placebo treatment (a "sugar pill" with no active ingredients, used on some trial participants, to help determine if using the treatment is effective—you'll learn more about this and clinical trials later in the book). Marcus decided not to try to get in the trial and instead see if he could get the experimental treatment. He reached out to the principal investigator (PI) for the clinical trial and received details about the treatment. Marcus then approached his oncologist with the information about the treatment and the contact information for the PI. His oncologist then went to the internal review board (IRB) at his hospital to get approval to give Marcus the experimental treatment himself. The board agreed, deeming the treatment compassionate care because Marcus's situation was dire, and he had little to lose.

Could you as a non-doctor with a life-threatening disease do the same? Yes—by sharing information about an experimental treatment with your physician. Even if you don't understand all the particulars of the treatment, the clinical trial team or principal investigator can help you communicate what your doctor needs to know.

When doctors are dealing with areas outside their specialty, they are confronted with many of the same obstacles non-physicians are: a lack of knowledge of the literature (and maybe even the vocabulary), current treatments, and ongoing clinical trials. Later in this book, you will learn about some of the resources physicians use and how you can understand the research that's being done or has been done—research that might help you to achieve the health outcome you are hoping for.

## Health Information Overload Is Real

The good news is that more than ever, determined patients and their medical teams can access helpful information. The bad news is that there is so much information out there that you as a determined patient need to let go of a fear of experiencing information overload and trust that you can sort it all out. Having someone who can help you take and maintain notes about your medical care can be invaluable if you fear becoming overloaded with information. However, even if it's just you trying to navigate it all, be assured that this book will guide you in getting to the information you most need to be an informed patient and strong self-advocate.

If it's hard for you to keep up on how best to stay healthy and manage any medical conditions you have, you're not alone. Over the last twenty years, the growth in health information has been exponential, as the chart below shows. In fact, over 1.5 million articles were published in medical journals in 2015 alone. Doctors and scientists can't possibly review all of this literature, which amounts to about 20,000 reports coming out each day, seven days a week! Physicians can only be familiar with a small amount of the total literature. They can't be up to date on everything. Even within their own specialties, it can be very hard to keep up. This is where you may come in as a determined patient with a very narrow area of health information that is relevant to you. You don't have to know everything; you just need to know how to access and make sense of research that applies to you.

Number of papers over time

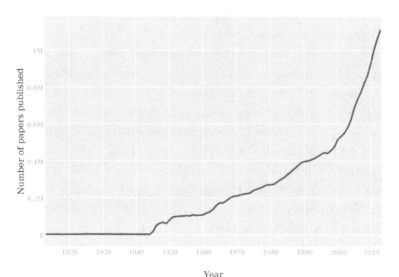

Year

We understand what you're experiencing. Together, we have been academic physicians and we are both actively practicing medicine. Dr. Danziger is running an NIH-funded basic science laboratory studying heart failure and hypertension; Dr. Gellens treated renal patients for many years and is knowledgeable in doing clinical trials on dialysis and renal failure. We have experienced firsthand the major shifts in how doctors and patients interact with each other in the age of information and how daunting it can be to find and focus in on the most important information for you in your unique situation. The explosion of disease-oriented sites and associations as well as books directed at patients reflects the changing landscape of health care: Pharmaceutical companies, hospitals, and medical clinics are marketing directly to you, the health-care consumer. But do you know how to sort through it all and not drown in conflicting and confusing information? When you consult your doctor and ask questions, do you know what to ask? Are you confident in asking for further explanation? Do you follow up with more questions if you're not completely clear about what you're told? Do you understand why certain tests or procedures are being recommended and others are not?

Maybe you follow health news and hear about new research studies. Did you know that they are sometimes misreported—and that you can look up most of these studies online and read them for free or for a modest charge? If you hear about a breakthrough and want to ask your doctor if a new intervention could be helpful to you, we have good news. We will teach you how to make sense of the research that was done and how to figure out whether it applies to your unique situation. Having fragmented knowledge about a particular condition and its common treatments isn't good enough and can lead to suboptimal care.

Resources change all the time, and thanks to technology, we'll see an increase in the number of options you have for quickly accessing the scientific and medical information you need to get a correct diagnosis and know your treatment options. We will also show you how to find the best health-care professionals and facilities for you (which may not be near your home).

By becoming a determined patient, you can make up for gaps created by the difficulties your medical team faces in managing the cases of hundreds of patients who have ever-changing conditions and needs. Customized medicine is becoming the norm, and it's important to begin looking at how to tailor treatments for you in your unique situation. Sure, you might end up doing exactly what your doctor prescribes. However, by researching on your own, you can feel much more confident in your decision to follow your doctor's orders.

We will teach you how to make the best of your visits to your physician (which are often very brief) by asking excellent questions about your treatment, including what tests and medications you need and how to avoid spending time and money unnecessarily.

## Partnering with Allies (Caretakers and Advocates)

As a determined patient, you should know that it's okay if you need or simply want someone to help you do research, be compliant with your doctor's orders, and find the motivation to keep seeking answers and help when your optimism is flagging. Your physician may be able to boost your confidence in your ability to get well but may not have the bedside manner or personal warmth you are seeking (later, you'll learn what you can do in this situation). Don't be afraid to ask for help from a friend who can come to appointments with you and take notes while you are emotionally processing what your doctor is saying. You might even want to work with a patient advocate who specializes in partnering with people like you. Ask your physician or a social services agency or your place of worship or community center if they know of any resources. Whether you partner with a friend or family member or you receive help from a professional advocate, remember that ultimately, it's your body and your health, so you will be the decision-maker. Your advocate's job is to help you, not tell you what you should do.

If you are helping someone who feels powerless over their medical care because of the complexity of the system, you can help that person navigate it and be proactive by reading this book and talking with them about best ways you can offer support. You don't have to feel helpless or passive and neither does the person who is looking to you as a caregiver or advocate.

We have seen many patients take charge of their health care and get the answers and interventions or treatments they need. We want you to become a determined patient as well, so let's get started with finding the right medical professionals for *you*.

---

## Notes on Becoming a Determined Patient

- If you feel you might not have gotten the correct diagnosis or a complete diagnosis, don't give up. Do more research and be willing to see one or more specialists.

- Doctors spend fifteen to twenty minutes on a typical appointment and see twenty-five to thirty patients a day. Despite time pressures, there are many good doctors who will take the time to answer your questions and who appreciate a determined patient—one who partners with their physicians to achieve the best possible medical care and health outcomes.

- No matter how effective the treatment, if you don't follow through on it, as directed, for whatever reason, it won't work for you.

---

- Come to doctor's visits prepared with specific information about your symptoms and with medical records. If you've had tests done, be sure you know why they were done, what the results mean, and what you are supposed to do after receiving any results that are negative or inconclusive.

- Be aware that while stress and aging are sometimes associated with mild memory issues and aches and pains, you do not have to simply accept a loss of health, mobility, or mental acuity. Leave no stone unturned in your quest for the best possible health.

- Consider subscribing to www.UpToDate.com or accessing it through a subscriber to learn about updates in recommended treatments for your condition.

- You may be able to join a medical trial or even access an experimental treatment in your quest to regain your health.

- You can better understand medical research and its application to you in your unique situation and discuss the new studies with your doctor and medical team.

- A friend, relative, or someone else in your community might be willing to be a determined ally and advocate, helping you to navigate the medical system and keep organized as you strive to improve your health and get the answers you need.

# DETERMINED TO PARTNER WITH PROFESSIONALS: FINDING THE BEST DOCTORS AND MEDICAL CARE FOR *YOU*

When someone's health isn't a big concern to them, any primary care physician they get along with well and who takes their insurance will probably seem good enough . . . but we know that's not the case for you. You want to find the best possible primary care physician for you—and you might need specialists or surgeons, too. Maybe your health insurance provider changed or you moved to a new location far from the doctors you trust, or maybe you are not getting better and you are questioning whether you're working with the right team of providers.

The bad news is that, like everyone, doctors are imperfect. Some are even incompetent or unethical or both, and there is less transparency about these doctors than there should be. Even so, we have good news. Many physicians are eager to partner with determined patients who are willing to play their part in bringing about the best possible health outcomes for themselves. You can become empowered to find great doctors for you given your unique situation—ones who will make excellent partners in your quest to maximize your quality of health. We're here to help you do that.

First, we want to help you learn more about doctors and their training so that you can better understand how to work with a team that might include a primary care physician, at least one specialist, and possibly surgeons, too. Good doctors know their limits and will refer you to a specialist when they feel you should be seen by a physician with more specialized knowledge and training in a particular area of medicine. Let's look first at the main doctor you will see—your primary care physician or provider—and then get into specifics about specialists and surgeons.

## Choosing a Primary Care Physician Who's Right for *You*

Not all primary care physicians are created equal, and in today's world, non-doctors—for example, nurse practitioners and physician assistants—are performing more and more of the functions of a doctor, serving as primary care providers. We recommend that if at all possible, you see a primary care *physician* because in general, this type of doctor has more training than a non-physician primary care provider does.

Primary care physicians, as they're often called, have at least one of two general medical degrees: an MD (medical doctor) or a DO (doctor of osteopathic medicine). An MD or DO is usually in charge of general medical care and refers patients to specialists as needed. Both follow similar undergraduate pathways with a bachelor's degree and pre-med courses taken before they enter medical school. MDs and DOs both take the Medical College Admission Test (MCAT), attend four years of medical school, and do a residency (paid training) at a hospital for three to seven years. During their residency, they have to do "rotations," meaning they have to learn about many different branches of medicine. That's why even an obstetrician will have some experience with cardiology and a cardiologist will have had some exposure to patients whose primary condition is mental illness.

Both MDs and DOs use the same methods of treatment, including drugs and surgery, and can practice in all fifty states as long as they have a license. However, a DO may place additional emphasis on the body's musculoskeletal system, preventive medicine, and holistic (whole-person) patient care, so these medical professionals have further training in these areas. MDs more often practice medicine in cities, suburbs, and larger towns; DOs frequently practice in small towns and rural areas. Also, DOs are most likely to be primary care physicians rather than specialists. Otherwise, all in all, DOs and MDs are equivalent.

Becoming a practicing doctor takes a long time. After completing medical school, all doctors do an internship, usually for one year. During their internship, they are known as *interns*, a term not to be confused with *internists*, who are fully trained physicians in their specialty of internal medicine and have passed their initial medical board exams in it. Doctors are required to retake their boards to renew their certification every ten years to ensure that they stay up to date with their skills and research. Physicians who are not yet board certified or who have lost their certification will typically be dropped from a medical group and have their hospital privileges revoked, so getting board certified and renewing certification promptly are very important in the medical field.

An internship is followed by a residency in a hospital, where the doctor in training learns by working in various specialties to get broad experience and a taste of what it's like to work in those areas. If doctors are especially drawn to surgery, dermatology, pediatrics, obstetrics, or something else, they might choose to become a specialist or a surgeon. As an example, Jay, one of the students in Dr. Danziger's medical school class, knew from day one that he wanted to do plastic surgery. He carved soap and whittled wood for fun, honing his skills in working with a knife. He studied every aspect of cosmetic surgery: why people choose to have it, how satisfied they are afterward, what innovations were on the horizon, and so on.

Not every aspiring doctor is like Jay, however. Some medical students make a very capricious decision when it comes to how they specialize. One of Dr. Danziger's best students on the internal medicine rotation simply decided that he did not like the personalities of those in internal medicine and liked surgeons better. Another student found out he did not like sick patients, so he decided to go into obstetrics, figuring that the patients would be happier when diagnosed as being pregnant rather than having cancer! Says Dr. Danziger, "I thought about going into ophthalmology since I thought that you could really (and almost instantaneously) improve someone's life significantly by restoring their vision through removing cataracts. And I was interested in how the brain processes visual information. The hours were good and the money quite adequate. It seemed an obvious choice for my specialty. However, once I did a rotation in ophthalmology, I realized two things: One, I did not have the manual dexterity to do eye surgery, and I didn't think that I could improve enough to be an excellent surgeon. Second, ophthalmologists are not interested in how the eye processes visual information in the brain. That was the domain of the neuroscientists. The first time I saw a human heart beating, I found it so fascinating that I shifted gears entirely and decided to go into cardiology. Although friends speculated that I went into cardiology because my father died of a heart attack, that had nothing to do with it."

Dr. Gellens initially was interested in geriatrics because she liked helping the elderly. However, she did a rotation that made her realize that she wanted to be an expert in one area instead. She loved learning about the anatomy and physiology of the kidney—plus, many of her patients with kidney disease were elderly. She ended up choosing to become a nephrologist.

The medicine residency, which helps the doctor in training decide on a specialty, is frequently followed by a fellowship of two to six years in a subspecialty. Doctors who serve as primary care physicians typically do a residency in pediatrics, family medicine, obstetrics and gynecology, or even geriatrics, which is a newer subspecialty.

During their time as interns and residents, physicians are in training but will typically introduce themselves simply as doctors. You can ask where they are in their training, but we will let you in on one giveaway that you are being treated by a medical student: Medical students usually wear short white coats as opposed to the longer ones worn by doctors who are no longer in medical school. Then again, when you're talking to a doctor in a long white coat, you may not recognize the limitations of their training and experience. You might need to be a bit of a detective to get a sense of the doctor's level of experience. You can always ask the nurse if you are hesitant to ask the physician. But it is important to know who is treating you and to know you can firmly insist, "I don't want a student doing that procedure," or "I don't want a student assisting with my surgery."

Dr. Danziger remembers that when he was an intern at the Mayo Clinic in Rochester, Minnesota, he met a patient who had traveled from Houston, Texas to Mayo because back home, the patient was getting conflicting advice on being treated for heart disease with prescription drugs versus surgery and wanted another opinion to help him make his choice. In Texas, the patient was seeing two of the most prominent cardiologists in the US: James T. Willerson and Denton Cooley. As Dr. Danziger says, "In talking to him, I realized that because I was working at the Mayo Clinic, he assumed I must be an expert. Meanwhile, I had been out of medical school for a full week! When he asked me what I thought about his case, I'm sure he thought I was more experienced." The right person to ask would have been the attending physician: the doctor in charge of coordinating the entire team. What's more, the doctors that patient was seeing back home happened to be the top in their field. Dr. Danziger had read their original research studies while in medical school.

Going to the Mayo Clinic or another well-known medical center for another opinion might be the right choice for you as a determined patient. We'll give you more guidance on that later in the book. For now, however, we want to be sure you know more about doctors and their training and experience so you can choose the right ones for you.

Your primary care physician should be board certified (or as doctors like to say, "have boards") in internal or family medicine or geriatrics. The exception is if you are a woman and want to use an obstetrician/gynecologist (OB/GYN) as your primary care physician, which is a common choice. We suggest your children see your family medicine primary care physician or a pediatrician, and again, these doctors should be board certified.

The difference between internal medicine and family medicine is the breadth and depth of the training. Family medicine doctors have training in pediatrics and obstetrics/gynecology and care for a variety of conditions in adults, such as diabetes or hypertension. On the other hand, internists have primary training in adult diseases and have spent several months in training focused on various specialties. If you want a single primary care physician who will take care of your whole family, you might decide to work with a family practitioner who knows everyone in your family and what is going on with them and their health.

One advantage of having a family medicine doctor is that they will be aware of what's going on with your family that might be influencing your own health. For example, from talking to your spouse, your doctor might know that your family's eating habits aren't the best. That might inform your doctor's line of questioning when talking with you as a patient. Keep in mind, however, that a doctor is required to protect each patient's privacy. Dr. Danziger remembers a patient who was married and worried that he had contracted a sexually transmitted disease from his lover—a concern this patient, understandably, didn't want to share with his wife. In a case like this, a doctor is going to do everything possible to encourage his patient to be responsible and protect both his sexual partners as well as himself. But if you're hiding your smoking habit or high cholesterol numbers from your spouse, your secret is safe with your family medicine doctor (or at least it should be because of HIPAA—Health Insurance Portability and Accountability Act—rules regarding confidentiality).

When choosing a new primary care physician, you might want an internist. Internists focus on learning about adult diseases and often have greater knowledge of these than family medicine physicians have, but internists might be harder to find in a rural area or small town. In fact, in some parts of the US, you might have difficulty finding a primary care provider who is a physician. You might end up with a nurse practitioner unless you are willing to travel quite a distance.

If you already have a primary care physician but are dissatisfied, know that you have the option of looking elsewhere—including outside of your health insurance network. When seeking a new provider, look for someone who understands where you are coming from, is accessible, has adequate experience, and provides quality care. What does that look like? A primary care physician should notify you right away if test results come back showing an abnormality. If they forget, it should be of concern. Calling in the wrong prescription or being insensitive to your feedback about any medications you're on and their costs and side effects are also red flags that it may be time for a change. A good physician should take a thorough medical history and ask questions to probe further into the details of your health—and should listen well. Doctors should pay attention to any signs that the underlying cause of your complaint is not the most common one. If you feel your doctor isn't listening when you point out what's different about your situation, including symptoms that aren't being accounted for, that's not good.

Often, patients wonder how much experience a doctor needs and might be uncomfortable with someone who appears to be new to the career. A colleague of Dr. Danziger's from the distant past was the youngest graduate of the University of Chicago Medical School. At twenty-one, he was a real-life Doogie Howser: a full-fledged MD. That was an impressive feat. But no matter how hard he tried to empathize with his patients, how professionally he acted, or how promptly he responded to questions, his patients were uncomfortable with his youth. He ended up growing both a mustache and a beard to look older and more experienced. If you have a choice and are more comfortable with a doctor who has not been in practice long, don't feel guilty looking into who else is available—but don't rule out "Doogie" without thinking through all the pros and cons of working with him compared to someone else.

You might want to ask friends whom they use as their primary care physician. If you do, ask them to be specific about why they like that particular doctor. Your friend might appreciate that the doctor is slow to prescribe medications when lifestyle and dietary changes could be just as effective in treating ailments. How comfortable you are with that attitude and approach might be different from your friend. Maybe your friend's primary care doctor is a family medicine doctor and you would prefer an internist. A brief meeting and interview before doing a physical or asking about specific health concerns can help you decide whether a doctor's a good fit for you.

Let's say your friend says his primary care physician is great, but your friend is twenty years younger than you are, runs marathons, and is in excellent health, whereas you're overweight and have recently been diagnosed with type 2 diabetes. Your friend's primary care physician might not be of great help in guiding you to live a healthier lifestyle when you have already tried your best. However, they could have tips and strategies you find very helpful.

## What Is a "Doctor" Anyway?

Lots of people can be called "doctors," including people with PhDs in art history and medical students on rounds at hospitals who are still in training and, as you learned, not yet licensed to practice medicine. Clinical doctors who can work in private practice, clinics, or hospitals are typically MDs, but they can also be DOs, AuDs, DPTs, and so on. Some people don't realize that if you meet a doctor socially, you might not be meeting a *medical* doctor but a doctor of philosophy (PhD) who is not qualified or licensed to practice medicine. Also, some doctors hold multiple degrees—even perhaps two doctorates.

Here's a simple way to think about doctors and medical practice: When it comes to being treated for a medical condition or physical ailment, you will be using an MD or DO. Without those degrees, a doctor can't prescribe medicine—except in a few cases, such as optometrists and podiatrists. That is why a clinical psychologist or an analyst you know as "Dr. Smith" is likely to have to send you to a medical doctor (such as a psychiatrist, who has an MD) to get a prescription for an anti-anxiety medication or an antidepressant. Their PhD or PsyD alone does not qualify them to write prescriptions, no matter how excellent they might be at providing therapy.

In selecting a primary care physician, check your insurance company's approved provider list, if you haven't done so already. Match these with any recommendations you are getting elsewhere (from friends, other doctors, and so on). Being affiliated with a teaching or university hospital is a good sign that a doctor stays informed about the newest research in his or her area.

You'll want all your doctors to be board certified, as mentioned, and you may want to check the state medical board to determine if there have been any disciplinary actions against a particular doctor.

Even the medical profession can be fooled by a physician's credentials, so don't be afraid to go to the website for your state's medical board and double-check that a physician genuinely is board certified. You can even go to the FBI's website to see their press releases on health-care frauds they've discovered. In a notable case, a "doctor" with an excellent set of recommendations from Italy was hired to do clinical research at the National Institute on Aging. His first task was to measure blood pressure while a patient was walking on a treadmill. When he did not appear to know how to use a blood pressure cuff or measure blood pressure, this "doctor's" supervisor became concerned and began to monitor him closely. After several months, he was fired. Using his "experience" at the NIH, he obtained a job as an anesthesiologist in another state. It was only after a patient died that it was discovered that he had never gone to medical school. However, the state medical board should have caught that.

In one of the largest fraud cases in New York, a man named Jose Katz employed unlicensed doctors to see and treat patients while billing under his Medicare/Medicaid numbers. Many conditions, most highly reimbursable, totaling $19 million in billing, were diagnosed. Katz and his unlicensed accomplices are now spending six and a half years in the same prison where Bernie Madoff was. While these cases are extremely rare, they show that in a busy world, it can be a good idea to double-check the credentials a doctor is claiming. The U.S. Department of Justice has an entire division dedicated to medical fraud, and their website has press releases on fraud that's been uncovered. It's worth looking at if you're wondering what kinds of behaviors to look out for. Sometimes the fraud is related to billing for services that weren't rendered, but sometimes medical professionals perform unnecessary medical procedures.

You can look up your doctor on the website of the American Board of Internal Medicine (ABIM), the American Board of Medical Specialties (ABMS), and other boards, such as the American Board of Family Medicine (ABFM), to assure yourself that they are currently board certified just as your insurance website or a health-care provider website claims.

Checking your own state's medical board to see if your doctor's license has been suspended or revoked or if there are any complaints or pending malpractice suits against that individual can be a good idea, but that level of research may not be enough. A recent investigative article by the *Milwaukee Journal Sentinel* and *MedPage Today* exposed the fact that when doctors move from state to state, their reputations may not follow them. While there is a national review database that has been around for decades— the National Practitioner Data Bank—it is incomplete. Worse, patients can't access it and may not know that a doctor has had many malpractice suits and complaints filed in another state. One of the examples the article cited was a doctor who had agreed with the Colorado Medical Board to "permanently deactivate" his license in 2014 but went on to establish a practice in Florida, which allowed him to be licensed even though he had complaints against him from seven patients in two different states. While the article reminds us that only 1 percent of doctors have patterns of multiple malpractice suits, the lack of consistency in reporting and making information available is disturbing. You might want to do an internet search to discover whether there are any states the doctor previously resided or practiced in, and then look into those states' medical boards' records. This advice holds whether you are working with a primary care physician or a specialist. We hope that what you find when checking up on a doctor is good news. If it isn't, you might want to alert your state's medical board to what you found.

## What You Need to Know about Referrals, Recommendations, and Reviews

Although any licensed physician with board certification should be competent, you probably want more than someone who is "just adequate." To narrow down the field of doctors to use, you can seek out referrals, recommendations, and reviews.

You can always ask other doctors you know for a referral. Doctors know other doctors both within and outside of their specialty. The pulmonologist who can't see you for a year might know someone who can see you within months. The podiatrist on your insurance list who is sixty miles away might know someone closer whom you could see. And if you have a limited network of doctors you are allowed to see, you could ask your insurance company about covering an office appointment with that podiatrist who is much nearer to your home. Your insurance company might have a website for looking up doctors by location, name, and specialty. However, one determined patient we know discovered that her insurance company had a PDF that she could print out or view on her desktop computer that had a much more comprehensive and organized list than the one she found on the website. If the "find a doctor" website is cumbersome to use, ask for a printout.

A primary care physician in a different group from the one you are in might refer you to a different specialist than your own primary care physician would. This may lead you to another doctor to check out. Sometimes, doctors have a choice of several doctors within a specialty that they refer patients to, and there might be a good reason why they always give out the same name!

When you're in the hospital or at a clinic and a specialist is assigned to you, it can't hurt to check that doctor's credentials before scheduling a follow-up appointment with them. The same is true if your primary care physician refers you to a specialist. Before making an appointment with the suggested specialist, you might want to ask your doctor this key question:

*Are you allowed to refer outside of your medical clinic or group?*

Dr. Danziger once had a lawyer in a large group who referred him to another attorney in the same group to help with a real estate transaction. This lawyer turned out to be incompetent and botched the case. Later, the original lawyer left the group and only then felt free to tell Dr. Danziger that his impressions about the other lawyer were correct. In the same way, sometimes, primary care physicians might refer you to someone who is not the best because they are required by the clinic or group that employs them to refer you to someone within that group. If you ask flat out whether your doctor can make a referral outside of the clinic or group, you might encounter a reluctance to give you a straight answer but go ahead and ask anyway. Your doctor's discomfort might be a sign of a desire to have more freedom to be honest with you—and a sign that you might want to do further research into the best specialist for you.

Do the basic research to make sure any specialist is board certified, takes your insurance, and is accepting new patients. If your insurance forces you to pay more for out-of-network providers or services, it's very important to check whether a doctor and the facility the doctor works at are in network for you. Keep in mind that if you do decide to see a doctor who is out of your hospital network, you might need to have an in-network doctor order any tests the out-of-network physician thinks you should have—that is, if you want your insurance to cover the costs of those tests.

Should an emergency come up at some point, the paramedics will take you to the closest ER, which might be at a hospital that is not in your insurance network. If you need to be admitted, it's best to find out if that facility is in network. The bottom line is that if you know you are dealing with a real emergency, get to an ER right away. Insurance companies are required to cover emergency services from out-of-network providers. But if you have a choice about which doctors and facilities to go to, know that going out of network might be very expensive for you—especially when it comes to tests and procedures not covered because the physician ordering them is out of network.

What if a specialist you want to see isn't taking new patients? You might want to ask if your primary care physician would be willing to make a call on your behalf to get you in. Sometimes, a nudge from another doctor will convince a specialist to make room in the schedule for you. Also, you could ask if the specialist is willing to see you if there's a cancellation.

You might have seen city magazines featuring profiles of the best local doctors, and those can be good places to search for a primary care physician or a specialist. Any doctor on these lists, which are put together based on recommendations by other physicians, is likely to be very good. It's important to know that some doctors are so busy and so focused on their work that they have no interest in getting their names into the rankings, so if your internist or specialist didn't "make the list," it could simply be that he or she didn't bother to try to get on it. The "Best Doctors in the City" list might be more accurately described as "A List of Doctors Who Went Along with This Themed Issue Because It Gets Good Newsstand Sales." In fact, some doctors simply pay to be on these lists, so it's important to know exactly what criteria were used to select the doctors who are being featured.

Another resource you might have come across is physician referral sites on the internet. Be *very* skeptical about these sites. They are fundamentally marketing services for physicians. Registration on the site will essentially give a doctor the designation of "five-star doctor" by Zocdoc, and the physician will be given an opportunity to buy plaques, mugs, and certificates to show anyone who looks that this doctor has been designated a "Top Doctor." These types of companies make their profits from the physicians who choose to list themselves, patients who subscribe to the service, and online advertisers. If you want to check these types of sites, ignore the doctor ratings and look at the reviews, while being very skeptical about their value, too.

Some have claimed that physicians post bogus negative ratings for their competitors. What's more, you can't know if the positive reviews were written by friends or relatives. This is especially true on sites where reviewers are allowed to be anonymous—you're relying on the site to verify that the reviewer actually was a patient.

To combat false reviews and manage reputations online, companies such as Reputation Defender and Demand Force have gotten into the doctor rating business. Their strategy is to counteract any negative reviews or ratings with a much greater number of positive ones they solicit. These might be genuine reviews, but do you completely trust companies that make their money by helping physicians clean up their online profiles?

## What Makes Someone a "Good" Doctor for You?

On websites for consumers that allow people to review doctors, the complaints often fall into the category of customer service, not medical help or diagnosis. It's not that such concerns aren't important, but they are probably not your priorities. You should have a doctor who delivers the best medical care, even if the waiting times in the office are long and the doctor's manner is gruff.

We personally know many physicians who are both very arrogant and excellent doctors. Perhaps they are arrogant because they know they are good. On the other hand, we know doctors who are egotistical *and* not good at what they do.

What makes a particular doctor "good" for you? Of course, you want them to be competent, but think about how flexible you might be able to be if you have to deal with someone who has a difficult personality. If you can get them to answer your questions and do more research on your behalf, or they help you make sense of research you've found, or they carefully monitor your health and how well treatment is working, do their personality quirks really matter that much to you? Ultimately, you have to be able to trust your doctor. If you don't feel comfortable with your provider, you are unlikely to get the highest level of care. You and your doctor have to be able to be honest with each other. A determined patient is careful not to take a doctor's attitude personally.

You can't change your doctor's personality, but you can insist on setting boundaries. For example, if your doctor jokes about your condition and it bothers you, you can say, "I get uncomfortable joking about my condition. Would you mind not trying to lighten things up with humor and just talking to me straight?" If the doctor seems impatient, you might say, "It seems like you're getting frustrated answering my questions, but it's important to me that I understand exactly what you are saying." Push for better explanations and for resources to learn more.

We know of a patient who was very nonconfrontational and embarrassed that she had trouble understanding her diseases. The patient's caretaker—her daughter—came to appointments and took notes. Sometimes, she would interrupt to make sure she and her mother understood what the doctor was saying. The caretaker noticed the doctor seemed a little embarrassed by how ineptly he was explaining procedures and how certain medications worked.

But after that, the doctor tried even harder to be clear in his explanations to his patient and her caretaking daughter.

If you think the doctor's ego is getting in the way of the treatment, or they're making you uneasy, ask questions about how they are acting and what you're being told. Call the doctor after a visit, if that makes you feel more comfortable. It's hard to feel confident and to question a doctor when you're in the examination room, especially if you're in a hospital gown!

If you feel judged or disrespected at any point in talking to a doctor, think about whether you will feel reluctant to confide in this person in the future. What if you develop a health challenge you find embarrassing or frightening? You need to be able to talk to your doctor about your health concerns and not fear that you'll be belittled or dismissed. After an experience that makes you wonder whether this doctor is really the one for you, by all means, start looking for someone else. However, if you don't have a wide choice of doctors, think about what your real objection is. Don't hesitate to move on from a doctor who writes the wrong prescription. The same goes for a doctor who ignores your medical history and prescribes a drug when it is contraindicated (meaning, given your medical history or your allergies to similar drugs, you should beware of taking it). A determined patient we know had a bad reaction to a particular antibiotic and brought it up to any doctor who asked about medication allergies or who wanted to prescribe an antibiotic, just to be sure that she never again had a serious, bad reaction to a drug that might be similar. If you follow your treatment and your condition isn't improving and you don't feel your doctor is concerned enough about the lack of progress, it is a sign to consider changing physicians.

When you have a medical condition, you are likely to see a specialist often, but surgeons are a different story. You'll probably have limited contact with them—except when you're unconscious in surgery! Does it really matter if they seem a little arrogant if you're only going to be in their office a few times?

Maybe you're worried that your doctor might react defensively if you're forthright in your concerns about them. As a determined patient, don't concern yourself with whether you hurt a medical professional's feelings or they become irritable or even somewhat rude because you're questioning the care you're getting. Your health comes first, every time.

## Interviewing Doctors

When choosing a doctor, you may be able to schedule a ten- or fifteen-minute interview appointment for little or no cost. You may end up working with your doctor over many years, so consider coming up with a list of three or so potential doctors and talking to them briefly in their office to see if you feel you could team with them easily. Let them know what you're looking for in a physician and why you're looking for a new doctor without going into great detail about what happened with the last one. The idea is to get across what your priorities are. For example, if you want someone who is open to your asking questions about new research you've read that applies to your condition, let the doctor know. Ask your doctors how they help determined patients achieve the best possible health outcomes. They might have tools you don't know about, such as being able to offer you easy access to your electronic medical records. Try to get a feel for whether these providers are good at communicating with their patients, staff, and partners in the medical clinic where they work (if they are working in a clinic); pay attention to any signs that communication mix-ups are common. Ask about how you would get help if you had a medical problem after hours. Ask, "At which hospitals do you have privileges?"

While talking to a specialist or surgeon, be sure to ask how many patients with your condition that doctor has treated and what the outcomes were. Doctors might be more forthcoming than you would expect in admitting they have little experience with a particular condition or ailment. A primary care physician might refer you to a specialist and a specialist might refer you to another specialist—or a subspecialist. If a doctor is confident about treating you, he or she should have no problem letting you know what the common outcomes are and what the worst-case scenario is. For example, let's say that someone with difficult-to-control hypertension is referred to Dr. Danziger for management of the condition. First, he will determine why this patient's blood pressure is hard to control. It could be that the patient is not accurately measuring their own blood pressure, is not taking the prescribed medications, is on the wrong medications, or has a secondary cause of hypertension, such as the narrowing of a kidney artery or a benign (noncancerous) tumor on an adrenal gland. It could be that the patient's body is resistant to known medications for the treatment of hypertension. The latter, coupled with a debilitating stroke or heart attack, is the worst-case scenario. The best is the first scenario: the patient was not measuring blood pressure correctly, perhaps because the blood pressure cuff was too small. It's even possible the patient doesn't actually have hypertension!

## At the Specialist's Office

When seeing a specialist for the first time, you will want to ask this key question: What's causing my symptoms or condition? There could be several underlying causes, and your doctor will probably want to narrow down the possibilities before suggesting a treatment.

You'll also want to be prepared to answer questions. That means taking with you notes on your health problems and, if it's a new doctor, your medical records. You might be able to have these sent ahead of time, too, but bring your own copies anyway.

The form doesn't matter. We've had patients show up with flash drives, CDs, and papers in manila files.

When your doctor wants to discuss test results and give you a diagnosis, bringing your spouse or close friend to your appointment might be a good idea. Having someone who can provide emotional support and perhaps even take notes when a lot of information is coming at you can help you remember all that was said and discussed.

To prepare for your appointment, refresh yourself on *why* you had certain tests or procedures done and what the results mean for you. The doctor will want to look at your results and be sure you understand what the numbers mean.

Often, making a diagnosis requires detective work and several tests. Each test result could be considered a clue that leads to the exclusion or inclusion of specific diseases or conditions. Eventually, if all goes right, adding up the clues means there is only one likely diagnosis. Even if this is not the case, it's common that several conditions call for the same treatment, so a final diagnosis is not required, just a narrowing down of possible diagnoses to a few. Determining the underlying cause is important if the symptoms don't go away with the treatment, however.

A specialist or surgeon should be able to give you some odds and numbers that can help you better understand the pros and cons and effectiveness of the treatment. For example, a surgeon might say to you, "I've done hundreds of these operations, and maybe 10 percent didn't solve the problem." If a doctor doesn't give you a direct, specific answer to your questions about the risks and effectiveness of the recommended treatment, and says something like, "These operations are done all the time," or "We have many patients with this condition and there's always hope," it's *possible* the doctor is hiding their inexperience. The idea is to find out how many operations *this doctor* has done and what the outcomes were—or what experience *this doctor* has treating someone with your disease or condition. Doctors can be overconfident in their skills and may think they can do a fine job treating you or operating on you, so they may dodge your question rather than be forthright. If you know they've only done an operation a half dozen times, you might want to get a surgeon with more experience. Be persistent and say, "I see. But how many operations have *you* done?" or "Okay, but how many patients with my condition have *you* personally treated?" Pressing for details is especially important for fully understanding the expected outcomes and risks involved, especially as per a specific provider.

Doctors typically prescribe standard treatments as determined by experts in the field, and you can read up on the most common treatments for your condition by using sites such as WebMD or the websites for national organizations related to your condition or disease, such as the National Kidney Foundation. Start here, and learn as much as you can from what has been written for laypeople. The websites for national organizations typically will let you know what treatments are on the horizon and what the latest research has found. Often, they will help you find in-person and online support groups, too, and you might discover that by communicating with other people who have your condition, you've got more questions to ask your doctors—and more research to do.

The truth is that you might end up having to see several specialists and getting a variety of tests and procedures to find answers. That's okay because as a determined patient, you will become empowered to find the best care! That is your goal. We believe that anyone with a medical condition should be proactive when it comes to taking charge of their health. If you have a condition that is life-threatening, leave no stone unturned in acquiring the information and help you need to get well. Any doctor should be glad to work with such a determined patient.

## Notes on Partnering with Professionals

- If you familiarize yourself with the various types of doctors, it might be easier for you to find a physician who has a lot of training and experience and who is right for you.

- Because reporting of malpractice suits and complaints against doctors is imperfect, you might want to research your doctor's reputation through your state's medical board as well as through the medical boards of states where he or she previously practiced. You deserve to know the reputation of a doctor who will be treating you.

- Your primary care physician may be under pressure to make referrals only to other doctors who are in your health insurance network ("in-network") or who work in the doctor's clinic. To access the best specialists, you may have to pay extra and do more research to find the best specialists for you.

- Do your homework when choosing a doctor and pay attention to any impressions you get when working with them. Be honest with yourself about whether a particular doctor seems resistant to your being a determined patient, and don't be afraid to try to change the relationship or switch doctors.

- If you received the wrong prescription or had your medical history ignored when a prescription was written, don't hesitate to look for a new doctor. You need to feel you can trust your doctor.

- Prioritize your health over feeling awkward about asking specific questions of a doctor. Be bold and ask how many times a surgeon has performed the surgery you're considering getting—not how many times it's been performed in the hospital or how common it is, but how often this particular surgeon has performed it.

- If you have a medical condition, begin researching it on the websites for the organizations related to that condition or to the system or organ that's affected—for example, the American Cancer Society or the American Heart Association.

## Chapter Three

# DETERMINED TO FIND ANSWERS: A ROADMAP TO RESEARCHING YOUR CONDITION

**B**eing diagnosed with a particular disease or condition can provide a sense of relief. Once you know what's going on, you can address your health challenge with the best possible treatment—at least that's how medicine is *supposed* to work. Not every diagnosis is correct and not every treatment is right for you.

A doctor might diagnose you correctly, but what if the treatment you are prescribed doesn't work as it should? Now you have a mystery to solve. What's really happening with your health and what, if anything, can you do to return to the state of health you were in?

If you sense that you are not improving, you could have the wrong diagnosis or you might respond better to a different treatment. Start with consulting a specialist, if you haven't already. And while your regular doctor will often be able to give you a correct diagnosis and recommend the best treatment for your condition, sometimes there is a person who responds better to another treatment that is less commonly used. When patients don't respond to the most common treatment for an ailment, they may have been misdiagnosed because they "almost" fit the diagnosis criteria, but further investigation revealed that they had a different condition or two diseases rather than just one to account for all their symptoms. In cases where the diagnosis and treatment are not leading to the state of health you want to experience or you are not improving as you think you ought to, you do not have to simply accept your situation.

You may have to see more than one specialist and do some of your own research into your condition and related conditions to get the answers you're seeking. Like Linda, you, too, might be having symptoms that are caused by a less obvious condition.

## When the Diagnosis Doesn't Seem to Fit

You might be misdiagnosed for a variety of reasons. The most common is probably that the doctor is focused on one unifying diagnosis that accounts for all your symptoms. However, sometimes a patient will have multiple problems that are independent of each other. For example, a person may have two primary cancers, such as one in the lung and one in the brain. The doctor might presume that one is primary and the other is a metastasis—that is, a tumor caused by the spread of the original cancer. This might cause the doctor to treat the cancer differently than if it were two separate cancers.

Sometimes, people are misdiagnosed because they don't report key symptoms that they've dismissed—and the physician doesn't think to ask about a particular symptom. If you've been under stress lately and having some issues with memory, your doctor or you might write off this symptom as the product of stress. But is that really the only source of your memory problems? When are you forgetful? What are some examples? Note them so you can talk specifics with your doctor.

Let's say you don't mention your recent forgetfulness, perhaps because you are embarrassed by this recent development, perhaps because you think it's no big deal. If during your office visit you're not asked if you've had any memory problems lately, and you don't mention that you have, you might be preventing your doctor from diagnosing you correctly. Maybe you have a condition that could be addressed with a new medication or a medication change.

Regardless of what your symptoms are, regardless of whether they make you feel embarrassed, note any recent changes not just in your physical state—pain, discomfort, shortness of breath, balance, and so on—but also in your moods, your energy level, and your mental sharpness. Make a point of recording how you are feeling and any discomfort you're having, maybe jotting down notes at breakfast each day when you take your medication or at night before you go to bed. Make sure you are ready with questions for your doctor if the symptom appears again.

If you've always had a certain issue related to a medical condition but your symptoms have changed—for example, they're becoming more frequent or more intense, or they're accompanied by another symptom, such as pain—pay attention and take notes. And if you've been taking a drug for a while, it's a good idea to look up its list of potential side effects to remind yourself of what they are. Some may be side effects you haven't experienced until now—and you haven't made the connection between the medication and what you've experienced recently. The medication might have overcorrected a condition, for example, and it's time for you and your doctor to reassess your medications.

When it comes to getting a correct diagnosis, keep in mind the old saying: To a hammer, everything looks like a nail. If you have back pain, an orthopedic surgeon, a rheumatologist, a general internist, and a sports-medicine doctor all might give you different treatments. Surgeons are likely to think about how surgery might benefit you, not because there are dollar signs in their eyes but because they think like surgeons and wonder: How can I fix this back problem with an operation? A rheumatologist might be thinking about reducing cellular inflammation to reduce the pain. Doctors have unconscious biases based on their training and experience. It's important not to accept a diagnosis when it doesn't feel right to you or it seems inadequate—for example, maybe you need medication *and* exercises. Research it further.

Earlier, you read about Linda's misdiagnosis. Her nurse practitioner assumed that an older woman with swollen feet had heart failure. Consequently, she didn't do extra testing or ask the kinds of questions that would have told her that something else was going on. That choice left Linda in discomfort, worrying about what was really going on and not realizing she was taking the wrong medication, which was causing inconvenient and unnecessary side effects. Steroids have some unpleasant side effects, too, but this was the best medication for her given that it could prevent her renal failure from getting worse.

You might end up having to see several specialists and getting a variety of tests and procedures to find answers. Knowing that every specialist may be biased (often with good reason), you can take charge and decide to get more information to be sure you are receiving the best care, advice, and treatment for what's really happening in your body. Then, you'll ask better questions of the specialists you consult.

Here's how it might work. Let's say you have back pain and aren't sure what type of specialist to see. You might have other symptoms as well that can give you clues about what your diagnosis is. For example, having skin nodules or joint pains in the small bones of your hands or feet can be a sign of arthritis. In researching your condition, you might realize that you have joint pain that you didn't mention to your doctor, and between your back pain and your joint pain, you actually have two symptoms of arthritis. In this case, you should see a rheumatologist. However, sooner or later you will probably end up with the correct specialist . . . it's just a question of how long it takes!

## The Differential Diagnosis

If you aren't getting relief from adhering to the treatment your doctor ordered, you might have been misdiagnosed, especially if you have more than one disease. Physicians are trained to try to find a single diagnosis that accounts for all the symptoms a patient is experiencing. They are also taught to make a differential diagnosis: They take a thorough patient history and, by process of elimination, narrow down the list of possible diagnoses. With so little time to spend with each patient, they can find themselves skipping questions that would reveal clues to the correct diagnosis. They might also forget to ask questions about symptoms that could reveal you actually have two conditions that are comorbid (appear together). They might have forgotten your family history that makes you more susceptible to certain conditions. They might not know about recent changes in your life, such as that you've adopted a new pet (that you turn out to be allergic to) or begun drinking more alcohol lately (and that is causing you to wake up in the middle of the night and have trouble getting back to sleep). Another example would be someone who is experiencing tremors because of both hyperthyroidism and early Parkinson's disease; that is, the person has two different diseases. Either of these could account for the tremors.

### *"Come to think of it . . . "*

Before talking to your doctor about a new symptom or health problem, it's a good idea to stop and think about what's changed in your home environment. Did you move to a new home where dust or mold might be coming through vents? Did you start using a new personal care product around the time you started developing a rash or redness? Has your lifestyle or routine changed? Are you eating more or less of a certain kind of food? Have you been taking new nutritional supplements that your doctor doesn't know about? Have you been exercising less often? Keeping a journal of when symptoms come and go can help you spot simple causes for aches, pains, and discomfort that you can easily fix.

Do not take self-diagnosis too far, however. At your next visit, tell your doctor what is happening—and make a call if your symptoms come back. It's wise to report all your symptoms to your doctor during visits, including when they appear and what their qualities are (for example, the type of pain, intensity, and so on). You will likely be handed a "review of symptoms" list, or your doctor will use one to ask you general questions about your health, such as whether you've recently had any gastrointestinal problems, shortness of breath, and so on. In preparation for a doctor's visit, you'll want to gather your own notes about your symptoms and perhaps, too, fill out and print a "review of symptoms" to remind yourself of any seemingly minor problems you've been having but forgot about. (You can do an internet search for a "review of symptoms" or "review of symptoms example" to find one.)

What if you report all your symptoms but your doctor tells you to just accept them, perhaps because they are common side effects of a medication you're taking or because your doctor feels these are causing you only minor discomfort or inconvenience and you should "suck it up"? That's when you'll want to do more research. You might have something going on that has yet to be diagnosed. You might have the wrong diagnosis. Or you might have the right diagnosis but benefit from a different treatment.

Tony's story is an example of paying attention to a symptom, talking about it with his doctor, and raising the issue again with a specialist rather than accepting that he would just have to tolerate it.

### *"That sounds like a statin."*

### *—Tony's Story*

Tony was referred to Dr. Danziger by a general internist to get greater insight into his cardiac conditions. The basics of his case were obtained from the referring physician, but Tony filled in the rest, which made all the difference. He said that he was a general contractor and he had recently developed a concerning problem his internist hadn't been able to help him with. Increasingly, Tony's memory was failing him: He was forgetting appointments, where he had left his tools, and so on. His internist didn't know what was happening and had ordered a battery of standard tests for dementia and/or "change in mental status" that included CT and MRI scans to look for brain tumors. The results were negative. Then Tony started researching the problem himself, using Google and a variety of websites. One was the Food and Drug Administration (FDA), which keeps a record of all side effects reported for each pharmaceutical drug for sale in the US. Tony wanted to know if his memory problems were in any way related to medications he had begun taking for his heart condition, high cholesterol, and high blood pressure.

He found that statin medications, which are used to treat high cholesterol levels, can cause memory loss. Tony looked up each of the medications that he was taking and found that one, Lipitor, was also called known as atorvastatin—in other words, it sounded suspiciously like a statin! His internist was familiar with the more common side effects of statins, including muscle aches and possibly diabetes, but didn't know of Lipitor's potential to cause memory loss, which was mostly reported in Europe.

"Do you think the medication is what's making me such a space cadet?" he asked.

Dr. Danziger asked him when his memory problems began, and fortunately, Tony could remember! They had started around the time he began taking the Lipitor for controlling cholesterol. It was the likely culprit—and he had been right in guessing that an atorvastatin was a statin. While Dr. Danziger knew of this side effect of Lipitor because he is a cardiologist, Tony's internist wasn't as well informed about statins as Dr. Danziger, which wasn't surprising since the primary side effects of statins that doctors look for are myopathies (muscle pains/cramps) and hepatic (liver) toxicity.

Now, thanks to Tony informing him, his internist knows about this side effect of Lipitor. He agreed with Dr. Danziger that Tony should stop taking the medication and try a different one to control his cholesterol that was not a statin and wasn't associated with memory loss. Sure enough, very quickly, Tony's short-term memory problems vanished and his cholesterol numbers were good.

It didn't take Sherlock Holmes to figure out what was causing Tony's memory lapses, but it did take information his internist did not have—and a proactive attitude on Tony's part. He came to Dr. Danziger's office prepared with good questions and his medical records, was forthright about what he was experiencing, and had done his homework, making Dr. Danziger's job very easy.

It's not always this easy to get to the bottom of what is causing a patient's symptoms, but as you can see, your research can help tremendously. With so much information available on the internet and access to that information sitting in your pocket or purse, you can become a determined patient like Tony—even if your case is more complicated than his turned out to be.

## Researching Diagnoses and Treatments

A search on the internet for your symptoms is likely to lead you to some good health websites, and you can go directly to them to do some searching if you are wondering whether your diagnosis is correct and fits your symptoms and whether you've been prescribed the best treatments for you. Here is a list of reliable health websites:

- www.WebMD.com and www.MedicineNet.com and their related sites

- www.mayoclinic.org or www.clevelandclinic.org, and www.hopkinsmedicine.org and websites for top medical clinics (including, perhaps, National Cancer Institute-designated hospitals and cancer centers)

- www.UptoDate.com (Later in this book, you'll learn more about this website, which is an important one for any determined patient doing research on a specific diagnosis.)

Start with these websites and work with your notes on your experience of symptoms to do some more searching. For example, Tony researched his medications and their side effects rather than just searching for "memory loss." Search for "knee pain" and you will get different results than if you search for "knee pain morning." Knee pain can have many causes, but knee pain that is worse in the morning is commonly associated with rheumatoid arthritis. If you have knee pain only in the morning, you'll want to mention this symptom to your doctor and ask for a referral to a rheumatologist, who can diagnose and treat rheumatoid arthritis.

Read up on the condition you think you might have. What are the symptoms to look out for? What are the causes of your condition? In some cases, you might be able to address those causes and overcome the condition completely. Failing that, you might be able to reduce your symptoms or halt them. Type 2 diabetes and prediabetic conditions are good examples. Diet and lifestyle changes can often reverse both.

When researching, use the websites we mentioned, but again, you also should look at websites for the national foundations or organizations dedicated to research and education related to that particular condition or disease. For example, you might want to spend some time on the website for the Arthritis Foundation if you are thinking you might have arthritis (or you've just been diagnosed). Websites for major US organizations devoted to the understanding, treatment, and cure for a particular disease or for diseases related to a bodily system (The American Diabetes Association, The Pulmonary Fibrosis Foundation, The American Heart Association, etc.) will also typically lead you to support groups in your area or online, such as conversation forums for people with the condition. They are also likely to feature articles on the latest research. All of that makes them good places to gather basic information. That said, you might want to go further in your research, particularly if your condition is very serious, you're suffering greatly, and/or you have a very bad prognosis.

At www.UptoDate.com, you can access the same information about your condition that your doctor is reading. It costs about $20 for a seven-day trial subscription, and you can cancel it afterward. Between the major medical websites and the ones for the national organizations for any particular disease or category of diseases, you'll learn quite a lot about your condition. UptoDate will likely fill in with anything new that hasn't yet been incorporated into the information available on the other sites, and the information is written in easy-to-understand language. Note that your physicians almost certainly subscribe to UptoDate because it is where they can read up on the latest treatment recommendations for various conditions and discover what changes to those recommendations are under review based on the latest studies. They—and you—can go to UptoDate to get the very latest on what's known about treating your disease.

If you're an especially determined patient, you'll consider checking with key opinion leaders (KOLs) who are doing the latest research on your disease. In Chapter 5: Determined to Turn Over Every Stone, you'll learn how to locate them and tap into what they know. For now, be aware that however frightened you might be by what you find on the internet, getting in to see a specialist sooner rather than later should be your next step, if you haven't taken it already.

If a specialist is booked up for many months, make an appointment, but be proactive. Ask the specialist to text or call you if any appointments open up in the meantime. Next, start checking to see if there are other specialists who can get you in to see them sooner. Refer back to Chapter 2: Determined to Partner with Professionals for strategies, and again, ask to be on the waiting list should someone cancel an appointment.

Also, if you spell out your situation to the doctor's receptionist, you might be able to get in to see the doctor sooner. All physicians build in some time off, and if your condition is very serious, they may be able to find a way to fit you in.

## When the Treatment Isn't Working

Even if you have the correct diagnosis for your condition, the usual treatment for it might not be right for you. Everyone's body is different, and you might be having a reaction to a medication that is more unusual and isn't listed among its known side effects. The surgery you had might not have eliminated the symptoms of the problem you and your doctor thought you had. You may have made lifestyle changes your doctor ordered but still find you're having the same old symptoms just as often. Fortunately, you're probably not having a unique experience—just one you and your doctor weren't expecting.

First, let's talk about medications as opposed to surgery. You can read a medication's insert or look up its list of side effects on the manufacturer's site or read about them on a health site.

However, you should also consider doing an internet search for the name of the medication and the term "side effect." People might be reporting side effects that haven't been officially recognized by the manufacturer yet. Be skeptical—people might be assuming the medication caused a particular side effect when, in reality, something else is causing a health issue. Additionally, if you developed any unusual symptom around the time you began taking the drug or shortly afterward, and you don't see it listed as a known side effect, it's important to do a search for that symptom and the name of the medication. Side effects can be underreported. Just because one isn't listed by the manufacturer doesn't mean someone taking the drug isn't experiencing it.

You might also check in with other patients who share your medical condition, using online forums or in-person support groups, to find out if anyone else has been experiencing the same problem. That can give you some anecdotal information that can help guide your research. Someone might already have identified that these two medications you're on can cause interactions when used together. If so, you'll want to talk to your doctor about possibly changing one or both of them.

Also, as soon as you take more than one medication, you could experience a side effect not associated with either one because the two drugs are interacting with each other. For a while, multiple medication pills were popular because patients were more likely to consistently take one pill than to take several. However, the compounds in a "polypill," as these medications are called, can cause symptoms the patient might not have had otherwise. Taking more than one medication can be cumbersome, but it might prevent side effects. (Plus, there are simple ways to remember to take your medications; see Chapter 4: Determined to Follow Through on Your Treatment to learn about products and strategies if you're having a problem.)

## Newer Isn't Necessarily Better

Clinical trials done before a drug is approved may expose several side effects, but what about any that show up after long-term use? These may not become known until you have been on the drug for years. A good example of this is "tardive dyskinesia," a spontaneous movement disorder that occurs after taking certain psychiatric drugs for a long period. When these drugs were first approved, researchers had not yet learned of this risk. Unfortunately, tardive dyskinesia is exceedingly difficult to treat and often permanent. One of the reasons an older medication might be a better choice for you than a newer one is that it's more established and the potential side effects for when it's taken alone or with other drugs are better known. It's possible that the new medication you've heard an advertisement for is as equally effective as other medications on the market but not superior. In that situation, it's especially important to remember that newer isn't always better and can even be worse (given the potential for unknown side effects).

It's common for some patients to have recognized a treatment side effect that hasn't yet been officially acknowledged by the medical community. The truth is that when a medication, type of surgery, or medical device is first introduced, long-term side effects may not have been identified. While the new treatment may seem to be better than the old one in some important way, patients are taking some risks in using it. As a determined patient, you need to weigh those risks.

What if a new drug is more difficult for the liver to process and leads to liver failure over time? What if a new treatment causes cancer or makes you more prone to certain types of hard-to-cure infections? You might end up feeling very fortunate that a new treatment or device was available to you, but before agreeing to it, as a determined patient, you should ask the same questions a doctor does.

## Questions to Ask about a New Medical Device or Drug Being Recommended to You

- What are the long-term outcomes? Does this device or treatment fail after a certain amount of time? Do the effects of the surgery last, and if so, for how long?

- Have there been any lawsuits against the manufacturer of the medication or device? Are there any pending? (Doing a search for the device or medication and "controversy" or "lawsuit" can help you answer this question, and you can check the FDA website, too.)

- Can I get the surgery reversed and any medical devices removed if that's what I want?

- What are the other options for addressing the problem? What are the downsides and upsides of those?

- Will there be any problems if I take this medication given the medications I'm already taking?

- Is this treatment my best option given my unique situation?

- What would you decide if you were in my position? Why?

The answers to some of these questions might not be clear yet. Maybe the studies done on a new treatment—for example, the use of an implanted medical device—only followed the participants for six months or a year even though the device would be expected to offer lasting benefits for the rest of the patient's life. The results might look very different if patients were consulted three years, ten years, or even twenty years down the road.

Stem cell treatment for heart arrhythmia, a dangerous condition that can lead to a heart attack or stroke, looked extremely promising once. Perhaps it still is, but the tried-and-true electronic pacemaker works well, and several stem cell research articles were retracted from medical journals after it was found that the results had been falsified. If the downside to the tried-and-true treatment is very burdensome or even dangerous, newer might be your best choice—but you should make the choice based on what is right for you, not on convenience or the desire to get that "cutting edge" treatment because you think it has to be an improvement on the old one.

The introduction of the blood-thinning drug Xarelto is a good example of the challenges in deciding whether a new medication is right for you. It's one of a newer class of drugs used to treat patients who have experienced blood clotting or who have atrial fibrillation, an irregular heartbeat that is associated with the development of blood clots. Blood clots can cause strokes that can disable or even kill you, so taking a blood thinner when you're at high risk for developing blood clots is almost always indicated. Traditionally, cardiologists have prescribed warfarin (which also goes by the trade name Coumadin) as a blood thinner to prevent blood clots and to treat atrial fibrillation. Take too little and you won't benefit. Take too much and you could experience another dangerous condition: a brain bleed or hemorrhage. Warfarin works by inhibiting clotting factors in the blood that require vitamin K to form. Thus, the effect of warfarin on clotting depends on vitamin K intake. Patients on warfarin have to watch their diet to be sure they're consistently eating the same amount of vegetables (the main source of vitamin K). They also have to work with their doctors to carefully monitor their blood and take the medication exactly as directed. No wonder doctors and patients were eager to consider newer medications that promised to solve these problems.

One of the problems with warfarin is that you need to monitor how effective it is in thinning your blood, or in medical terms, how it affects your international normalized ratio (INR), a measure of how thick your blood is. Monitoring requires being seen by a visiting nurse or getting to a clinic or lab regularly. If you're on a blood thinner, you typically have to visit your doctor's office once every couple of weeks to have your blood drawn. For you, that might not be such a big deal. For someone else, it may be a major inconvenience.

The drug Xarelto was introduced as an alternative to warfarin and works through a different mechanism. Xarelto was marketed as easier and more convenient to use because unlike warfarin, the INR does not have to be monitored constantly. If you live a two- or three-hour drive from a lab where you can have your blood tested, you might think, "That's the blood thinner for me!" However, it turns out that Xarelto needs to be taken two to three times per day to ensure there's enough in your system to prevent clotting but not so much that you have excess bleeding. But Xarelto was marketed by the manufacturer as a "once a day drug" presumably so that it would be as convenient to take as warfarin (which is taken once a day). Research showed that if you take Xarelto once a day, the amount of the drug in your system would frequently start too high, leading to excessive bleeding. There is now talk of a class-action suit against the manufacturer. It might turn out that Xarelto is a better drug than warfarin when taken more than once a day, but it was marketed as providing the benefits of warfarin without patients having to undergo frequent checks of their blood as they do with warfarin. Now that you know that Xarelto doesn't seem to work as promised, you might be doubtful of future claims made by the manufacturer.

Clinical trials may not reveal all the side effects of a drug, as noted. You should know that you'll be helping others if you report to your doctor your own side effects and unusual symptoms you believe might be associated with your medical treatment.

If you are on one medication and are experiencing a side effect that isn't listed anywhere, go beyond just doing a search and reading any anecdotal evidence on forums, which isn't of great value.

Go to the FDA website and look to see if anyone else has reported it as a side effect and report it yourself after talking with your doctor (who surely will want to know what you're experiencing and talk it through with you). If you're taking more than one medication and having some unexpected side effects, same advice. It's possible that a different drug or drug combination would be better for you. If your doctor says, "None of my other patients have a problem with this treatment," remember: Your body is unique, and you might be in a small group of people who don't respond well to a treatment that works for most people.

All of us can take heart in knowing that more and more, we'll be seeing customized medicine—testing before a prescription is written out to determine which drugs are likely to be better for you given our unique DNA. You might need a different drug, a different formula, or a lower or higher dose. Communicating with your doctor about your experiences with a medication is vital if you're to achieve the best possible health outcomes for you. If you are taking a potentially life-saving medication, such as an anti-depressant or a blood thinner, it's all the more important not to stop taking your medications or even taper off them without being medically supervised.

## When the Lifestyle Changes You Make Aren't Enough

Let's say your team of doctors and you decided you did not need to go on medication or have surgery for your condition, but the lifestyle changes you have made haven't had enough of a positive effect on your health. Your doctor might talk to you about medications and/or surgery at this point. However, if you're a determined patient, you will be honest about yourself regarding compliance. The truth is that patients often intend to make lifestyle changes but face obstacles. For example, for many, losing weight is exceedingly difficult. It may be of value to enlist an expert who can help you—a dietician or nutritionist, for example. You might want to work with a counselor or even a weight loss coach to discover and address any psychological roots to your challenges with losing weight. Maybe you might want to join a group like Weight Watchers or Overeaters Anonymous, or use an app or software to keep you on track with your health goals, or change your grocery shopping, cooking, and snacking habits as well as your exercise habits (for example, adding weight training). It may be, too, that your lifestyle changes are helping but not enough, in your opinion—and perhaps your doctor's, too.

If losing weight will alleviate your knee pain, and despite a serious effort, you're not losing weight and your knees ache, that's worthy of a conversation with your physician. Maybe you need to get occasional steroid shots or take steroids orally for your knee pain or take pain medication or some combination of the two for now while you schedule knee replacement surgery. You might consider weight-loss surgery before getting knee replacement surgery. Your doctor can help you decide what the best option is for you, but not if you're hiding the truth about what you're doing and experiencing.

When you see your doctor, explain what you've tried to do to change your lifestyle—what did and didn't work and why. Should you feel judged, speak up during the appointment or afterward. It's okay to need extra time to process your emotions before expressing to your doctor that you're not okay with the words, facial expressions, and tone of voice used when talking to you about why you weren't able to lose the weight you wanted to lose.

Let's say you're taking medications but considering surgery. Be frank with your doctor about your medication use and whether you're complying with your doctor's orders 100 percent. No treatment will work if you don't follow through with it. If you don't take your medications as directed, talk with your doctor about why that is to see if together, you two can come up with some solutions to the problem. In the next chapter, you'll learn about how you can achieve better health outcomes by being better at complying with your doctor's orders. Being honest with yourself and your doctor about what you are doing between visits is key.

## Notes on Finding Answers about Your Condition

- When a treatment isn't working, you might have an incorrect diagnosis. If you haven't seen a specialist, see one now.

- Observe and record your symptoms so you don't forget the details: Record the time of day you have them and note their intensity and qualities. Note any lifestyle changes you've made or experienced lately. Bring your notes to your next doctor visit.

- You may have to see more than one specialist to get diagnosed properly.

- Consider researching side effects of your medications that are not included in the official list of known side effects. Manufacturers might not yet have identified and listed newly discovered side effects. If you take two drugs or more, you might experience side effects that aren't listed for either medication.

- Check reliable medical and health websites to learn more about your disease or condition. Then, consider subscribing to and checking www.UptoDate.com to learn the latest recommendations for treatments.

- Newer isn't necessarily better when it comes to treatments.

- Be honest with your doctor about any challenges you're having in making lifestyle changes related to your health condition.

# DETERMINED TO FOLLOW THROUGH ON YOUR TREATMENT: BEING HONEST ABOUT "COMPLIANCE"

In this new era of physician and patient partnership, we wish there was a better word than "compliance" to describe how well you follow your treatment plan. If you tell your doctor you'll stop smoking but don't, or that you take your medication but secretly, you skip some doses, you're not being compliant.

The truth is that compliance isn't always easy. You might have obstacles to following through on your doctor's orders that you're not entirely comfortable discussing, or you might just get frustrated by how hard or inconvenient it is to undergo the treatment and skip it. Even so, as a determined patient, be honest with your doctor about what's happening and why.

Your doctor isn't an authority figure to be obeyed by a compliant patient. Those days are over. Good physicians will listen to your concerns and consider changing your treatment if you're struggling to follow it. However, they won't know if compliance is an issue unless you are forthright with them. Don't let guilt or embarrassment get in your way. To achieve the best health care and the best possible health outcome, you need to be determined to set aside any emotional discomfort or other obstacles to doing what you need to do to get better.

Why is following through on your treatment protocol vitally important? In some cases, not being compliant results in a treatment being only modestly effective, if that. In other cases, it can lead to serious problems.

Dr. Danziger's cardiology patients often are on blood-thinning medications after receiving a stent for coronary artery disease. These drugs need to be taken for at least a month (and frequently, for years) to prevent the stent from clogging (also known as "occluding"). If the blood-thinning medication isn't taken daily, the patient is more likely to suffer a major heart attack. That's why cardiologists will consider a patient ineligible for a stent if they believe the person won't take their blood-thinning medications as prescribed. If you struggle to remember to take your pills, or to buy them, or you don't like the side effects of your blood-thinning medication so you skip it sometimes, be honest with yourself and your doctor. As a determined patient, you can work with physicians to come up with a solution that will work for you—and it may be surgery.

Why don't people simply do what the doctor tells them? Cost can be a factor.

## Getting the Best Prices for Tests, Procedures, and Medications

It's unfortunate that in the US, many patients are expected to do comparison shopping for health care even when they're sick or in pain. However, at least some medical care can be delayed while you compare costs. Knowing how you can determine what you will be charged for procedures, tests, and medications, and how your insurance works, can help you be more assertive when you are in an emergency room, clinic, or hospital. You don't want to get stuck paying more than you have to for recommended procedures and tests that you can schedule for a time that's convenient for you. When you need medical testing done and you're not in an ER or checked into a hospital, you might not want to automatically use the nearest and most convenient lab if you will be paying some costs out of pocket. One patient found that routine blood tests done down the hall from his specialist's office cost double what a self-standing lab would charge.

That said, your doctor might have a preference for what lab to use based on how accurate they've found the lab to be over the years, but talk with your doctor about the costs if you're concerned. Some doctors have no idea what the lab they're sending you to will charge you for a particular test. Others will know the cheapest, most reliable testing facility that's near you.

If you're consulting with physicians out of your network or who don't take your insurance, let them know if you have had recent tests whose results you can send to them or upload to a medical records site they use rather than having the tests repeated. One determined patient kept a copy of her blood tests from when she applied for life insurance and showed them to her doctor at her next checkup. With these results entered into her electronic records, the doctor didn't have to order duplicate tests for which she would have had to pay because she had a health insurance deductible.

Because of legislation passed at the end of 2020, health care providers will be required to provide you with costs, making them available on a website for example, but until the law goes into effect in 2022, you can ask them for the "private pay" price and the price they will charge if you use your insurance. You can also comparison shop for nonemergency testing through sites such as http://www.NewChoiceHealth.com, http://health.costhelper.com, and http://www.ClearHealthCosts.com to get a ballpark figure of what testing might cost. Sites such as these rely on patient self-reporting and provide an insight into what insurance companies and health-care providers often aren't sharing with patients.

Generally speaking, you'll have an easier time learning the costs of medical procedures by speaking with someone in the provider's billing department than if you speak to your insurance company. If you can, learn what the codes for specific procedures are or are likely to be (a doctor can't always know ahead of time all the problems that will arise during a procedure and all the codes that cover those complications). A determined patient is not afraid to ask what the possible codes are for a procedure before agreeing to it and being billed for hidden costs associated with particular codes. For example, let's look at a common test, a colonoscopy, that, according to federal law (the Affordable Care Act), is covered by your health insurance at no cost if you are fifty or older and you have never had a colonoscopy before. You might be surprised to know that there are many different codes for colonoscopies—for example, there's one for a screening of someone at average risk for colon cancer and a different one for a screening of someone at high risk.

Here's how things can go wrong. If you've been having digestive problems that might be signs of colon cancer, the procedure could be coded as a diagnostic colonoscopy. If you're due for a colonoscopy according to the rules of the Affordable Care Act, and your doctor asks, "Have you had any digestive problems lately?" and you say, "Come to think of it, I've had some constipation in the last few months, probably because I've been traveling a lot and not eating as well as I could," in theory, your doctor could order a diagnostic colonoscopy (but probably wouldn't, knowing that you're due for a free one anyway). A screening colonoscopy in which polyps are found and removed might be coded differently than a screening colonoscopy in which that wasn't the case.

Ask your doctor what happens if polyps are found while you're under anesthesia. Will they be removed and biopsied, or will you have to come back to have that done? Whenever you're going to go under anesthesia, you should speak to your doctor beforehand about what will happen if the exam (or surgery) doesn't go as you both hope. Everything has a code, and if you don't want surprises, ask questions before you get the procedure, assuming that's possible. Of course, once you receive a bill, you can ask your insurance company to question codes you believe are incorrect. Billing and coding mistakes are common, so if you're paying a bill, make sure you know every item on it.

The site https://coder.aapc.com/search/ will identify codes for various treatments. You can also learn about specific codes by going to https://www.findacode.com/cpt-code-set.html and signing up for a free trial so you can look up specific codes and their explanations.

You could ask your insurance company what will be charged, but they might not tell you. Some insurance companies are required by providers to not disclose costs, having signed a legal contract called a nondisclosure agreement (NDA). When you start your research on costs, ask the provider, "What is the price if I use my insurance and what is it if I don't?" They might quote you two different prices.

You might decide it's easier to wait until after you have agreed to a procedure and you receive the bills or notification of what your insurance company was billed for and what your portion of the bill will be. But knowing what your options are for having frank conversations can help you to avoid hassles with bills after you have had medical treatment and should be focusing on your health, not making sense of bills. If a close friend or relative asks, "What can I do to help?" after hearing you've got some medical problems, you might want to consider asking them to help you go through your bills and contact the providers and your insurance company. Medical billing is complex, and it's common for bills to have errors. If you have a deductible or coinsurance, catching those mistakes might save you money.

One of the most common causes of sticker shock for patients is using an out-of-network physician or facility. As a determined patient, you will want to be aware of which doctors, clinics, and hospitals are in your network and what it would cost you to go out of network to get treatments and consult with physicians. You can try to negotiate with your insurance provider to see whether they will treat an out-of-network doctor as in-network, but there are no guarantees that you'll get both parties to agree on a fee you find reasonable given your deductible and coinsurance. But it makes sense to try if there is no specialist in your network, or the only one is many miles away, or the only ones in network aren't appropriate for you for some reason, or the specialist who has been treating you suddenly is no longer in network. Start with having your primary care physician make your case for you *before* you get treatment.

Too often, health insurance policies cover mental health care while the number of mental health care professionals within their network is tiny—just one example of how you might have services covered in theory but not in reality. If you are self-referring to a physician or other health-care professional because there truly isn't an appropriate provider near you that is in network, we encourage you to find out what you need to do to get the physician's services covered—even if just partially. Be sure to keep a paper trail and follow up with any instructions the insurance company gives you. If you're told, "We'll call you back on Tuesday," note that promise on your calendar. If you've heard nothing by the end of Tuesday, call back the individual you spoke to. Getting an individual's complete name and direct phone number, as well as the name of their department and even their title, can really help. You don't want to linger on hold for forty minutes only to get a vague promise of a call back that might or might not happen.

What we're telling you might seem obvious, but it's common for people to feel reassured by someone on the phone and then forget to follow up. When it's just a matter of having to make a phone call and tell someone your story all over again, it's simply inconvenient. If it's a matter of not being told that your test results came back and some of the numbers indicated a possible problem, or you were supposed to get a call back on an appointment but never did, your health might be compromised.

Let's say you do get a call back from your insurance company and they tell you they have denied your right to see a specialist, have a procedure, or get a test and have it paid for despite your doctor's recommendation and referral. It could be that on appeal, your insurance company decides to go with your doctor's recommendation after all. Ask your doctor to call them again.

If costs for a surgery, testing, or treatment are going to be unaffordable for you, you might want to upgrade your insurance to keep the price of surgery and postsurgical care down, assuming you can put off surgery. We know of a patient who needed a knee replacement and switched her insurance plan to one that offered greater coverage in exchange for a higher premium, but she was in significant discomfort while waiting for the window for changing her plan.

Increasingly, determined patients concerned about costs are considering medical tourism. Traveling out of the country to get surgery, have a procedure or test done, or buy medications opens you up to the possibility that you won't have an advocate with you if you have a complication with a procedure, which might make you feel uncomfortable. But there are also many health-care providers outside of the US who will give you care equal to that which you would receive back home.

Some people do medical tourism for reasons beyond the high cost in the US—for example, they might want to have a pleasant vacation while getting dental work done at half the cost. But regardless of why you're considering medical tourism, do your research on having a procedure there versus here. Ask about how many follow-up visits are needed (if any) and how long you should stay in the country after surgery. What happens if you have complications, such as an infection or excessive bleeding? Even simple operations can go wrong.

Will you be up for a very long flight home once you're released from the hospital? Are you ready to do all the planning and checking involved in setting up your trip and changing it if something goes wrong with surgery?

Think about whether you would feel comfortable getting an operation in a foreign country where yes, the staff speaks English and the facility is accredited, but you don't have a companion who can come with you to be present when you wake up after surgery, advocate for you if something goes wrong, and accompany you home after you're released. It might be easier for you to have someone play this role for you if you stay closer to home.

Increasingly, insurance companies are providing incentives for patients to get surgery done abroad. One East Coast insurance provider flies people to Mexico for knee surgery that will be done by a US surgeon who will also be paid to fly in—and the surgery is provided at a major hospital. If you're seriously considering medical tourism for a procedure, do your homework. You might want to check out the guidebook *Patients Beyond Borders: Everybody's Guide to Affordable, World-Class Medical Travel* by Josef Woodman and Jeremy Abbate.

Some people might say that buying medications out of the country is a form of "medical tourism." Some patients will make a special trip to another country to purchase pharmaceuticals or devices such as asthma inhalers, glucose testing strips, or EpiPen auto-injectors—or when they're traveling, they'll make a point of buying these items. Some medications can be purchased from Canada using online pharmacies, as long as you have a prescription.

The law has not come down hard on individuals buying small amounts of medications or medical devices out of the country, but please talk with your doctor if you're thinking of going this route. You can't necessarily trust what you're getting. Law enforcement has found some pills marked as having been manufactured in a particular country when they were actually made elsewhere. If the package isn't truthful about the origin of the medication, what other truths might be hidden from you as the consumer? Weigh the risks when deciding to buy medications or devices from non-US sources.

## Why Stretching Medication Isn't the Way to Go

Too often, patients will cut pills in half or ration them to save money on medication. If you're thinking of doing this, talk to your physician. You want to be in compliance with your doctor's orders, and you might not realize it, but compliance might mean taking tablets whole, not splitting them in half.

In other words, let's say it's cheaper for you to buy thirty 6-mg tablets than it is to buy sixty 3-mg tablets and your doctor wants you taking the 3-mg pills. In some cases, you can split a 6-mg pill into two 3-mg halves using a pill-splitting device available at a drugstore and not suffer any consequences, but many medications don't work as well if you break the tablet's coating.

On the other hand, if you're taking one tablet rather than two—that is, half a dose rather than a full one—you're not adequately following through on your doctor's treatment. Discuss with your doctor the challenges you're having taking your medications exactly as prescribed. You might have options you don't know about—for example, different sized pills or alternative medications, or a cheaper source for your prescription drugs. Always talk to your doctors before changing your medication regimen for any reason.

Also, don't hesitate to ask your pharmacist about your medications. These professionals can often answer questions and offer suggestions you can take up with your doctor. They might even call your physician on the spot to ask a question about the prescription.

## Inconvenience You Just Can't Tolerate

Inconvenience can be a factor in patient compliance, too. If driving across town twice a week to do testing is driving you crazy and you're starting to miss appointments for tests because it's too hard to time the traffic, talk to your doctor. There might be a closer facility, and you might not need to have so many appointments after all. Consider, too, that you might have transportation options you aren't aware of. A local senior center or community health clinic might be able to alert you to a transport service that can reduce some of your burden. If the side effects of a medication are so inconvenient and undesirable that you find you're not taking the medication, think about how you felt before you started using it. Dr. Gellens has patients who understandably don't like spending hours in a dialysis center undergoing kidney dialysis only to feel very fatigued afterward. Skipping dialysis has long-term and short-term effects, so she counsels them on their options to make sure that they comply with her prescription for regular dialysis—whether at home, which is not only possible but preferable in some cases, or at a dialysis center. A drug might cause you to feel fatigued, but again, there might be options you haven't considered.

## Addressing Forgetfulness

Starting a new habit is easy, but maintaining it can be hard. If you're like most people, you probably need some tricks to jog your memory so that you take your medications or do your exercises as directed. One of the easiest things to do is to attach reminders to a wall by your nightstand or where you store your medications.

(Hint: If you store them out of sight, find a better place than your bathroom. The heat and moisture from showers and baths can affect the medications, so it's better to store them in a clean, dry place—or, in some cases, your refrigerator. In fact, some drugs are meant to be stored in a refrigerator.)

Having your medications out in the open, maybe on your kitchen table, can help, too, but be careful if you have young children around or they sometimes come to visit you. You might prefer not to have childproof caps, which can be hard to open, but in that case, you have to keep your medications far away from children. Then, too, while you might not want to believe it, someone you know might take your pain medications or medications that can alter mood or be used to create street drugs. Get rid of medications you are no longer using by dropping them off at a safe medication drop off, whether it's your local pharmacy, a police department, or someplace else. Don't flush unneeded medications down the toilet because they can affect the water supply. Let professionals who know how to safely discard them take care of getting rid of your extra pills.

Do you forget to take your medications because you're disorganized? That's common. Maybe you take a lot of different medications or have an erratic schedule. You might need to start taking a medication at night but forget because you've never taken pills at this time. Aside from leaving the medication on the nightstand, you can also set an alarm that reminds you to take it. You can also try smartphone applications and software that will not just cause a mobile phone to ring or buzz but send you notifications about why the phone is ringing or buzzing.

If you find it hard to read the type on medication labels, come up with a system to counter that. Keep a pair of reading glasses by your medications so you're sure to read the label every time rather than assuming you grabbed the right vial. Put a big bold sticker on the top of the vial that says "2 at Bedt" (meaning "take 2 at bedtime").

Finally, having support can help you get past the obstacles to following through on your doctor's orders. You might want to join a support group for people with your specific disease. And if you're a caretaker, try to be aware of how difficult it is for even the most determined patient to be perfectly compliant. Together with the person you're helping, maybe you can come up with some ideas that can make things easier.

## Following Through on Instructions Before and After Surgery

If you and your doctor decide you need surgery, you'll be given preoperative and postoperative instructions. Take them seriously. Lifting something heavy after cataract surgery can lead to a detached retina and another surgery. Not telling your physician that you had a snack the morning surgery was scheduled could result in serious complications on the operating table. Don't take chances. Pay close attention to the symptoms that are signs you need to call your doctor, even if it's in the evening or on the weekend.

### Eliminating Three Common Communication Barriers

To be a determined patient, you'll want to be sure that whenever your doctor gives you instructions, you listen carefully and read any written instructions thoroughly. If you still don't understand, ask questions. Sometimes, however, even if you're trying your best to understand, there is some sort of communication barrier getting in your way.

1. *Language.* The most obvious communication barrier might be that you and the doctor don't speak the same language, literally. In this case, a translator can serve as

a bridge, and most hospitals have translators who can speak languages common in the community. If you suspect your accent or a speech impediment is getting in the way of being understood, ask for a piece of paper to write down what you are saying. Never be embarrassed by a language barrier. There is no shame in having someone who is more fluent in English or is more easily understood accompany you to your appointment. And if you have trouble understanding your physician's accent, don't be embarrassed to ask them to say something again or rephrase it.

2. *Hearing loss.* Your doctor might not realize your hearing isn't the best or that you have trouble focusing on important information your doctor is telling you when there's a lot of background noise. Don't strain to hear. Speak up and get to a quieter space where you can talk more easily (or, if you're in a hospital or clinic room, ask for the doctor to close the door and speak more loudly).

3. *Understanding medical and visual/spatial concepts.* Ask about definitions of medical terms and whether your doctor knows of videos that can help you understand a medical concept such as how a particular medication works at a cellular level or how a heart pumps. Your doctor might also know of videos that demonstrate exercises you need to do postoperatively. Some people have trouble mentally picturing visual/spatial concepts and find videos that show systems in three dimensions much more helpful than two-dimensional illustrations or photographs.

Determined patients don't hesitate to make sure that medical information, instructions, and guidance are crystal clear to them.

If you're a patient and not following through on your treatment as you know you should be, ask yourself: How important is it to keep doing things the way you have been compared to achieving the outcome you want—better health? How is being inconsistent in your follow-through affecting your health, your energy, and your everyday life, including your interactions with your family members and friends? What are the payoffs to being a determined patient and leaving no stone unturned compared to being halfhearted about managing your health condition? As physicians, we can't take your medications for you or drive you to the clinic, but we can encourage you to find every possible way to do what you need to do to achieve the best possible health outcome.

---

## Notes on Following Through on Your Treatment

- Don't let costs get in the way of getting the medical treatment and testing you need. Assume there are alternative options that you can afford. Talk with your doctor, insurance company or Medicare or Medicaid, and the provider to get the information you need to help you access health care.

- If navigating the complexities of your medical bills is stressful and time-consuming, consider getting someone to help you with this so you can focus on your health.

- Cutting tablets in half, which breaks their coating, can make many medications less effective.

- Consider ways to make accessing medical care and complying with your doctors' instructions more convenient and a "no-brainer." Routines can help with taking medications.

---

- Always follow all the after-surgery instructions you're given and call your doctor if you have any concerns.

- Communication barriers can get in the way of good health care. Don't let embarrassment stop you from finding effective ways to talk with your doctor so that you understand what you're being told and your doctor is truly taking in what you are saying.

## Chapter Five

# DETERMINED TO TURN OVER EVERY STONE: BROADENING YOUR RESEARCH

L ifestyle changes, medication, surgery—all can help you manage your condition and maybe even return to a state of health you enjoyed previously, as long as you continue to follow your doctor's orders. However, you might find yourself frustrated by the difficulty in making the lifestyle changes you and your physician agreed upon. The side effects of the medication you're taking might be significantly reducing your quality of life and causing tremendous inconvenience. Surgery might not have produced the results you hoped for. Thanks to the internet, you can cast a wide net when it comes to researching the latest ways to treat your condition— and any conditions you might have that you didn't know about. For example, you might not realize that it's common for people with your condition to suffer from depression or anxiety, sleep disturbances, and digestive disorders. Is it your medication that's causing the problem, and if so, are there alternatives? Do you need other medications but haven't realized it yet? You can broaden your research into your health with the help of experts in a particular area of medicine and through looking at what clinical trials are starting up, ongoing, and have recently completed but whose results have not yet been published.

You can also try to get input on your case from top medical centers and key opinion leaders.

## Working with the Top Medical Centers and Key Opinion Leaders (KOLs)

When you have a very poor prognosis, you might want to book an appointment at the nearest top-rated medical center. That could mean Mayo Clinic in Rochester, Minnesota; Cleveland Clinic in Cleveland, Ohio; or Johns Hopkins Medical Center in Baltimore, Maryland. It could also mean the nearest top-rated medical center for your disease that is highly ranked by *U.S. News & World Report* or a National Cancer Institute-designated cancer center. If you don't have a bad prognosis but simply are frustrated that the specialists you have seen locally aren't helping you achieve a treatment plan that works for you, you might want to check with top medical centers, too. Before you call for an appointment or prepare for a road trip, however, you will want to do as much research from home as you can.

You might decide to identify key opinion leaders (KOLs) and contact them. These are individuals recognized by others in their fields as the top experts, aware of the latest research and theories about how particular diseases will be prevented and treated in the future. They are frequently sought out by pharmaceutical companies for their opinions and views on both new and existing agents/treatments.

KOLs are also busy researching medical conditions and very often can be found working at major medical centers, where they share what they have learned with those centers' teams of clinicians who treat patients. However, sometimes these individuals are not affiliated with the top-rated hospitals for a particular disease. They might not see patients, but they could help answer questions for you about whether the research they are doing might help you in your situation. Contacting one could be invaluable if you have a rare disease or a very poor prognosis, when taking the risk of undergoing an experimental treatment may have far more upsides than downsides. A KOL sets up a research study or leads the team and can help you decide whether it's worth trying the treatment despite its experimental nature and its known side effects. However, if you want to know which researcher to contact about a particular study, you can do an internet search for "key opinion leaders" and the name of your disease—for example, "key opinion leaders pancreatic cancer"—to see what comes up. Another good place to start is to check the "corresponding author" listed in an important research study. If the author can't answer your questions, you can ask to be put in contact with the KOL who led the research team. (Later in this book, you'll learn more about research studies that are worth paying attention to and trying to read yourself.)

If you feel uncomfortable calling a total stranger to see if that person can help you, remember, as long as you've done your research and aren't completely unfamiliar with that KOL's work, they will probably be happy to talk to you.

Let's say you think you might want to get an appointment at one of the best hospitals for your condition, such as an eye disease. Do your research to find out whether some KOLs are on staff there. Maybe they simply have high-quality specialists and you'd like to get examined by at least one of them. According to the *U.S. News & World Report* list, the best hospitals for ophthalmology are the Bascom Palmer Eye Institute, Anne Bates Leach Eye Hospital in Miami, Florida; the Wills Eye Hospital at the Thomas Jefferson University Hospital in Philadelphia, Pennsylvania; and the Wilmer

Eye Institute at Johns Hopkins Hospital. But let's say you live much closer to the Mayo Clinic in Minnesota. You might go to the Mayo Clinic, which is lower on the rankings but still listed. However, knowing who the key opinion leaders are when it comes to your particular eye disease can help you decide which ophthalmology department to contact for an evaluation. Note that if they are willing to see you, it might take some time to get an appointment, and the office visit and any testing done on the premises might not be covered by your insurance, but they may have the expertise you need to get the answers you're seeking.

The trick to finding a KOL is to do an internet search for the most recent studies done on your particular disease. A search will take you to the sites previously mentioned but also to research studies, particularly if you use Google Scholar (https://scholar.google.com/) or PubMed (https://www.ncbi.nlm.nih.gov/pubmed/) to do your searches. The first or last name listed is that of the head researcher. If you find articles on a study, it's likely that the journalists interviewed the lead researcher to get a quote summarizing the findings of that person's research and how those results fit in with other research that's been done. And you'll see the same names coming up again and again as you pull up more studies on your condition.

Once you have the name of a KOL who researches your disease, you can look them up. Where are they doing their research? Are they attached to a hospital where you can be seen by clinicians who are likely to be very aware of the new research in their specialty? That's typically the case, but sometimes, the KOL has gone into private practice or left the university where the research was done.

You can contact KOLs directly and ask about their research and how it might apply to you and your situation. A KOL will probably be glad to share with you names of any clinicians they know of who are both treating patients and aware of the other

KOLs doing groundbreaking new research in the area. Researchers and KOLs don't generally work alone. They work in groups and attend national and international meetings together. They know each other and what they are doing scientifically.

If you're a really determined patient, you might attend a scientific meeting on your disease. If you want to do this, be sure to pick the right one. Some are more clinically based, so researchers present studies on clinical trials, whereas others are more focused on cellular and animal studies. You might want to see which studies are going to be presented and who is presenting them, as the speakers are likely to be key opinion leaders.

Practicing physicians who have a lot of experience in treating patients with a particular condition might be willing to see you and consult with you even if they can't take you on as a patient given how many people they're already treating. They might even be willing to consult with you by videoconferencing.

If you have a team of physicians near your home who are monitoring your care, the KOL or members of the team of clinicians at another hospital might be willing to talk directly to your doctors at home with your permission. Using the expertise of professionals far from home as well as the ones nearby, you can assemble the best possible team to help you as you manage your disease or condition and strive to improve your health. Talk with your local doctors about how to make this happen.

Let's say you choose to get a second opinion from another expert in the field of medicine in which your disease falls (and that can be a very wise choice!). After receiving the second opinion, you have several options. You might want to switch your care to the physician providing the second opinion or ask the physician providing the second opinion to work with your primary doctor. Alternatively, you could just listen to what the doctor with the second opinion has to say. If your case is complicated, your best bet might be for the two physicians to consult with each other in deciding your best treatment. Sometimes in an academic medical center, a division will convene a conference to discuss a single patient. This commonly happens when an individual's case is complicated and therefore interesting to the physicians. If it does, you are certainly free to ask to attend—and you can mention to your doctor that if they will be attending a conference on your health, you would like to be present to learn more, if that's okay.

As for understanding the research that's being done, when you don't have a medical or scientific background, making sense of it all can seem daunting at first. Your doctor can give you the basics on your condition and the disease process, but the next chapter will help you get a better handle on cutting-edge research that doctors know how to access. You can develop a better understanding of the results of ongoing and recently completed clinical trials that have been reported in medical journals as well as the results of any research that might drive future clinical trials, such as experiments on mice and on cells in petri dishes. What's coming down the road may give you a sense of hope and optimism, both of which can help you to keep working at doing your research, getting the help you need, and managing your condition.

## Clinical Trials and You

Most people have heard that getting into a clinical trial can give you access to experimental treatments that may turn out to be key to regaining your health or improving your condition. That can be true, but it's important to know how they work.

First, clinical trials have different phases:

In phase 1, researchers determine the short-term safety of a medical device or a drug and observe the bodily responses. Do the participants' conditions improve? Worsen? Remain the same? Phase 1a trials of medications are for determining safety (stage 1a), and phase 1b is for determining proper dosage (stage 1b), which is related to safety but to effectiveness, too. Phase 1 trials tend to have very small numbers of participants.

In phase 2, the efficacy of the drug or device is tested in up to several hundred people now that its safety is better established. These phase 2 trials are often randomized and controlled, meaning one group is given the treatment and another group (the control group) is not. These may be blinded studies, meaning the patients don't know whether they are in the control group or the treatment group. Phase 2 trials of medications can also be double-blinded; neither the patients nor the researchers know which patients are in the control or treatment groups.

A phase 3 study is performed if results from the phase 2 are promising in showing a beneficial effect of the treatment (note that about one-third of new drugs are successful in phase 1 and 2 studies). In phase 3 drug trials, the medication is tested against a placebo (a pill that has no active ingredients) or against another drug in several hundred to thousands of patients.

A phase 3 study can take up to several years to complete and be properly reviewed, which can be frustrating for patients and doctors seeking medical breakthroughs. However, phase 3 studies are very important because they provide greater understanding of the effectiveness of a treatment. Superiority is determined in phase 3 of clinical trials. If a drug proves to be just as effective as one that is already on the market but it is more convenient—for example, you only have to take it once a day rather than three times—that could be considered a quality that makes the new drug superior to the old one. But if it has worse side effects and costs the patient considerably more out of pocket, is it truly superior from your point of view as a determined patient? Remember, newer isn't always better.

Once phase 3 is completed and the results show that the new medication is an effective treatment, a pharmaceutical company can apply to the FDA for approval to market the drug.

This process, including the clinical trials, can cost hundreds of millions of dollars, and it helps explain why new drugs can be extremely expensive.

In phase 4, a drug or medical device already approved by the FDA and on the market is studied over a long period to evaluate the long-term effects of taking it. These trials can uncover more information about effectiveness, safety, and side effects.

If during some phase of a clinical trial researchers can see that a drug is clearly not effective or that some trial participants experience unanticipated, serious side effects, the trial will be halted. For example, in the 1990s, a large trial on hormone replacement therapy (HRT) on menopausal women was stopped when the researchers realized participants getting the HRT were at increased risk of blood clots, cardiovascular disease, strokes, and breast cancer.

Participating in a clinical trial might not help your health condition at all, it could make it much better, or it could make your health worse. Researchers are vigilant about the latter possibility and will call off a trial if they have evidence that the experimental treatment is harming participants.

Even if you get accepted into a clinical trial you apply for, remember, the treatment is still likely to be very experimental. For non-placebo studies, researchers have to rely on statistical analysis and, in the case of medical devices, imaging studies to be sure the treatment is safe and effective. For example, redesigned insulin pumps and artificial joints are studied by having patients use the devices and report to the researchers who are gathering information. Researchers' data can help determine whether a "new and improved" version of a device is any better than the old one. You can also check the FDA's site at https://www.fda.gov/medical-devices/medical-device-safety to read recent announcements about medical device safety based on both the FDA's monitoring and patient reporting. Note that you can also report any problems you've had with medical devices on this site, too.

Many devices are now supposed to be able to work with apps, but the communication between the device and the app might not work as well as advertised, so check with your doctor and the FDA to be sure that the app isn't giving you false reassurance. Also, some security breaches have been discovered with apps. You might not be worried that someone will hack into your insulin pump and change the settings, but because this can be done, the FDA's website has a warning about the cybersecurity risk and information about what you can do (replace the pump with a more updated version).

If you are in a clinical trial involving a placebo and think you're getting the new medication that is being tested, your mind might trick your body into responding as if you were actually receiving a helpful medication. Also, a physician who knows which patients are getting the placebo and which are getting the medication being trialed might, without realizing it, cause patients to realize which group they are in. That's why during clinical trials of medications, researchers use a double-blinded process—they make sure the patients have no idea whether the pills they are taking are placebos or the medication being studied and that the doctors are "in the dark," too. (This is why they call it a "double-blind" or "double-blinded" study.) The drug and the placebo—and the older, established medication, if that's part of the study—are made to look exactly alike. In addition to designing the study to be double-blinded, researchers will use statistical analysis to be extra sure the placebo effect didn't taint the results.

Your participation in a clinical trial can move research forward by helping the medical community better understand what treatments do and don't work, so you might want to participate in the trial even though you might not experience any benefits personally. Then, too, sometimes the trial is of a lifestyle-related treatment or treatments. A clinical trial of using yoga versus meditation versus simply taking time to do relaxing activities to reduce tumor growth doesn't have many downsides.

Thus, when it comes to clinical trials of medications and surgeries, you might want to think about whether you want to simply continue with your treatment as the doctor ordered or look into using the experimental treatment or surgery yourself— assuming that you can find doctors who are cooperative and the downsides are minimal. If you have stage IV cancer, you might be more open to an experimental procedure or drug—and you might be able to access it. In any case, you'll want to know what clinical trials are ongoing. If nothing else, you might feel more hopeful knowing that every day, researchers are working hard to find better treatments for all sorts of diseases and conditions. A breakthrough may be in your future.

## Finding Clinical Trials You Might Benefit From

To find a clinical trial, you can go to www.clinicaltrials.gov. Your doctor and a national organization for your diseases might know about them, too, but clinicaltrials.gov is the best, most up-to-date resource. You can learn which trials are still seeking applicants to participate and which are ongoing. If a trial is ongoing, you need to see if they are currently recruiting patients and, if so, whether you meet the criteria for participating.

If you can't get into a clinical trial but your prognosis is very bad, you might be able to receive an experimental treatment not as part of the clinical trial but by qualifying for what's known as "compassionate care"—your doctor can make the case to a hospital or clinic team that you are entitled to try an experimental treatment given how little you have to lose. Compassionate care treatments are almost always approved.

Increasingly, researchers are mindful of the differences between people who are cleared to participate in a clinical trial and patients who are seeking new and better treatments. Clinical trials involve patients who agree to the inconvenience of participating in the study. That eliminates a certain number of people—including people who might fit your particular demographic. In the past, much medical research was performed on white men, and it was assumed that the research would apply to any other adult. For example, a study of the antidepressant medication Zoloft showed it to be very effective for the male participants. However, later studies showed that Zoloft is not nearly as effective in women. Similarly, clinical trials showed that Ambien was more effective than a placebo at helping men who suffered from insomnia. Later research showed that women metabolize Ambien differently than men do, so doctors need to consider lowering the dosage of this medication if prescribing it to a woman rather than a man.

Are you the same gender and age of the participants of a particular trial? Could the participants' lifestyle have affected the results? When looking at a study, keep these variables in mind. Consider, too, whether the study was of people who only have one medical condition—for example, heart disease or diabetes but not both. If you have a second medical condition, your body might respond to the treatment differently.

If you do want to participate in a clinical trial, be honest with the researchers when they ask about other conditions you might have. They want to keep the results as reliable as possible. Ask plenty of questions about the commitment involved. They might want to track you for several years. Will you be able to return to the medical center to continue doing the trial even if you move? Can you report in from your new residence if you move away while the trial is ongoing? If you're given the green light to participate, stick with the protocol exactly as it is spelled out, but communicate to the researchers and your doctor about any new health problems that come up. They might or might not be related to the experimental treatment, but you help yourself and potentially other patients in the future by being observant of and reporting on what you're experiencing as you undergo the treatment.

## Notes on Broadening Your Research

- As a determined patient, you might decide to research treatments for your condition that are newer and that your medical team might not know about or recommend. Educate yourself about the limitations of promising research and how clinical trials work before discussing alternative treatments with your doctor or doctors.

- If your health situation is very dire, you might end up contacting a corresponding author of a research study and even a KOL (key opinion leader) who designed the study about a particular experimental treatment to ask about whether the treatment could save your life. You might be able to access the treatment even if you don't participate in the clinical trials.

- You can work with a local team of doctors and a team at a larger medical center so that you can access the most up-to-date specialists and key opinion leaders.

- Clinical trials are conducted in phases, and early trials focus on safety, whereas later trials focus on safety and effective dosages of medications. The further along in clinical trials a medication is, the more likely it is to be an effective treatment.

- Double-blinded or double-blind clinical trials are the most reliable type of clinical trial because the placebo effect—the mind's ability to affect outcomes—could taint the results otherwise. If you participate in a clinical trial of a medication, you won't know if you're getting the placebo. If you participate in a trial of a medical device, you will know whether you're getting the device being tested.

- When researching clinical trials, recognize that you might not fit the demographics of the participants. This is true whether you're researching ongoing trials or trials that have gone through all the phases.

# Chapter Six

# DETERMINED TO UNDERSTAND: THE BASICS OF READING JOURNAL ARTICLES ON RESEARCH

As you are learning about your diagnosis and treatment, you will probably start reading materials written for laypeople to get the basics. You can begin with WebMD or the sites for organizations dedicated to your disease or condition, such as the American Cancer Society. However, truly determined patients take it a step further, learning the latest information about their disease and even reading actual research studies rather than just summaries of them. The more you know, the easier it is to manage your disease or condition, be sure you are getting the best possible treatment, and better partner with any medical professionals on your team.

Relevant articles are generally broken up into two types: basic studies (on cells, insects, and animals) and studies on people (such as observational studies, clinical trial studies, and longitudinal studies). There are also studies of studies (meta-analyses of basic studies or studies on people). Let's look at each of these three types.

## Basic Studies

Basic studies are done in laboratories and often involve experiments with biochemicals and cultured cells (cells grown in a laboratory). Experiments are commonly done "in vitro" (Latin for "in glass"), so an in vitro study looks at what happens in a test tube or a petri dish. The next level of basic research uses insects such as fruit flies, which have a short life cycle so you can easily study several generations of the insects that have been treated, or it uses live animals, whose anatomy is more similar to humans—think rats, mice, and other rodents, and sometimes, but rarely, monkeys or apes. While some have raised ethical concerns about doing experiments on animals, these types of studies can provide researchers with valuable information on disease processes, prevention, and treatment in humans and inspire the setting up of clinical trials on humans. That's because animals can have many of the same diagnoses, symptoms, and prognoses as humans. Because of genetic engineering and screening of animals used in experimentation (rats and mice, for example), scientists have learned a great deal about diseases ranging from heart failure and hypertension to pulmonary fibrosis.

Consider a recent study done at Rutgers University using mice, called "Combinatorial treatment of idiopathic pulmonary fibrosis using nanoparticles with prostaglandin E and siRNA(s)." The research showed that in mice in which the lungs were altered to be similar to those with the lung disease pulmonary fibrosis—that is, a mouse model of pulmonary fibrosis—the treatment used in the study reduced mortality and lung damage in the mice, which inhaled very small particles (nanoparticles) of certain substances (prostaglandin E and siRNAs). If you had idiopathic pulmonary fibrosis and you did not qualify for a lung transplant, and despite taking the currently approved medications, you were seeing your condition deteriorate, you might want to show a new study like this to your physician to learn whether you might be able to access the treatment. You would do this knowing that what happened to the mice's lungs might not happen to human lungs, however. You would want to go to www.clinicaltrials.gov to see if there is a clinical trial of these treatments being set up or underway. Of course, you would want to know the potential downsides of any experimental treatment offered to you as compassionate care. But again, when your prognosis is very bad, you are likely to accept risks you wouldn't accept if it were a better one.

Knowing that there may be new treatments down the road can help you to be optimistic, but it's important to understand that no matter how promising the results of a particular study or clinical trial are, the results may not be reproducible. Irreproducibility of research has become a major source of concern for the scientific community. According to a 2016 article in *Nature,* 52 percent of over 1,500 researchers surveyed said they felt that reproducibility was a "significant crisis," which is understandable: "More than 70 percent of researchers have tried and failed to reproduce another scientist's experiments, and more than half have failed to reproduce their own experiments." That might be distressing, but the good news is that 41 percent of medical researchers say that in the last five years, their labs have made improvements that could increase the reproducibility of study results.

If the study was not flawed, why can't other researchers perform the same or a similar experiment and achieve the same results as the first study? We don't always know, but the answer can range from poor experimental design to normal biological differences (variability) among participants to unconscious bias (for example, the pressure to publish positive results can cause researchers to unknowingly downplay negative results) to outright fraud. What we do know is that when studies can be reproduced and the same results achieved, that's typically when standard treatments will change. Until that point, even the most promising study has to be seen as offering hope but not reliable guidance. Also, individuals respond differently to treatments—some respond very well while others may not respond at all and still others experience mixed results. Clinical trials help determine who, if anyone, responds and how.

## Studies on People

Observational studies offer insights into what's happening with patients being treated by medical professionals—for example, in a particular clinic. They can arise as a result of doctors observing certain patients achieving better outcomes or groups of patients unexpectedly developing a comorbid condition (that is, another medical problem). By looking at the medical records and data, with the patients' permission, doctors can share what they're observing, adding to the body of medical knowledge and potentially inspiring other studies that lead to changes in recommended treatment protocols.

Longitudinal studies are types of observational trials that look at groups of people over a long time—or look back over historical records. Longitudinal studies often find correlations, such as a connection between smoking and heart disease. These types of observational studies can be difficult to conduct and usually involve a lot of people, and some will drop out over time. Consequently, there aren't as many longitudinal studies as we might like. Still, the ones that have been done have advanced the body of medical knowledge. One example is the Framingham Heart Study which began in 1948 with over 5,000 participants, which taught us about connections among diet, exercise, and cardiovascular disease. Thanks in no small part to this longitudinal study, we know that people who rarely exercise have a higher risk of developing heart disease.

## Studies of Studies

Review articles and meta-analyses combine the results of many similar studies. Review articles summarize the literature on a topic while meta-analyses combine the data and results of several studies. Meta-analyses are often performed when conclusions from various small studies conflict with each other, providing clarity about how to interpret all those results. Because meta-analyses look at the results of many different studies, including ones on patients who have very different profiles from you, you have to read them carefully to discover any specific studies and conclusions that most closely apply to you in your unique situation.

## Where to Start Your Research to Find Studies

It used to be that research studies were only available in printed medical journals that physicians subscribed to—for example, the *New England Journal of Medicine* and the British medical journal the *Lancet*. These and other well-known journals can be found in many libraries, particularly medical school libraries, which also subscribe to more specialized journals such as the *Journal of Cardiovascular Risk* and the *American Journal of Nephrology*. When the internet came in, access to studies became much easier for everyone. Anyone with an internet connection could find articles through a simple search of PubMed or Google Scholar—and that's still true today. You might be able to access a full article for free, or you might only be able to access the abstract unless you pay for the entire article. If you're having trouble getting to the complete article, you can ask at a university, college, or medical school library what they would require for you to access journals via their subscription. You might also ask a friend who has privileges at that particular library to help you out.

Journals generally have the most up-to-date information, right out of the laboratory, which is great. And access has become so easy that determined patients might come across and read a new research study before their doctors do! But where do you start your research?

In addition to using Google Scholar or PubMed, you can simply type "research" and some keywords (such as the name of your condition) into a search engine. Some sites about research, such as www.ScienceDaily.com, give laypeople brief overviews of what's being published in medical journals, so you might want to start there. Each article has a link to the original study. Wikipedia might give you an overview of a study or a condition, but just like with any site that summarizes and interprets research, you will probably want to click through links to the actual research.

You might also hear about studies from the media, from organizations devoted to health and perhaps your specific disease or condition, and from sites for major medical centers or publications. Check UptoDate to see if the new research is mentioned or has affected treatment recommendations or might in the future. As you do your research, you may find that the same research articles are interpreted differently by journalists and writers for websites. In this case, looking at the actual studies can help.

## "What's In It for Me?"

Whenever you hear a news story or read an article on a particular condition or disease, including how to prevent it, first, it's important to pay attention to whether the study was on people like you: for example, adults over fifty, people who have medical conditions like yours, women as opposed to men. If you're doing caretaking for a child or older person, you'll want to look at whether there are studies or specific recommendations for these groups—and you'll want to discuss the studies with pediatricians or geriatric specialists.

As mentioned earlier, keep in mind your gender, age, medical conditions, other medications, and lifestyle choices as well as your genetics, such as any diseases that run in your family.

Medicine is becoming more customized, and in the future, it will become easier to know how established and new research applies to individuals. That is good news for everyone. You may have heard recently that the medical community has discovered that many women who underwent chemotherapy for breast cancer did not benefit from it. Chemotherapy has some very bad side effects—including reduced immunity. People have been known to die of the flu or colds after having had their immunity compromised by chemotherapy. Consequently, oncologists are now being careful to personalize the treatment of breast cancer, checking patients' genetic profiles, to make sure their patients receive the best possible treatments for them. When talking to your doctors, always ask if there are any genetic tests that can help you make decisions about medications, surgery, and medical devices.

Have you been diagnosed with more than one disease or condition? Consider that when looking into research. Studies done on a new medication might not have involved participants who had both conditions, and you might want to wait for more research before trying the new drug.

As you are looking at a study, consider, too, whether the downside of the new treatment is so small it may be worth making a change in how you're managing your disease. A study showing that yoga or meditation reduced migraines may not be very reliable because it's the first study of its kind. But if you take up yoga in the hopes of reducing migraines, that might not be such a bad choice! If using a certain medication three times a day instead of once a day promises to yield better results, you and your doctor might decide to try out a new medication regimen as an experiment. However, even if want to make what seems like a harmless change in how you are managing your condition or disease, you should always discuss it with your physician. Your doctor might know of some potential downsides you should factor into your decision—or have some good advice about how to make those changes.

## Is the Research Reliable?

Once a study has been completed, researchers write up their study design and results and submit the article to medical journals. This is the way most new medical information is disseminated to the medical community. Often, the same results are also presented at medical meetings.

Before an article is accepted into a medical journal, it is peer-reviewed. That means that other experts in the field read the article, ask questions, and offer suggestions that could improve it. There may be some bias to the interpretation of the results or a flaw in the statistical analysis that is worth pointing out. The authors have a chance to edit the article to address the feedback and then submit a new draft.

The better research journals have several layers of experts in the field who review articles submitted for publication. The more thorough the review process, the more reliable the journal and the studies it accepts for publication. The editors of these journals don't want to be embarrassed by publishing a study that has flaws because their reputation and the journal's are on the line. Occasionally, articles are even retracted—and having layers of reviewers helps the editors of journals feel more confident that the research studies they publish were done properly and yielded valuable results.

When they review a study or article for publication, experts in the field are looking at the following:

- How new the information is
- The technical quality of the work
- How valid the study's claims are considering its results

- Whether standards of research in the area were upheld by the research team

- The quality of the data and whether the math (the statistics) was done correctly

- Any ethical concerns related to animal or human subjects involved

Researchers around the world submit their articles to journals in their home countries, and this research will typically get discussed at medical conferences. Sometimes, studies from countries outside the US will appear in English-language medical journals and in English-language articles in the media.

Traditional media outlets such as CNN, the *New York Times*, the *Wall Street Journal*, and medical centers that offer health news—such as Harvard Medical School and Mayo Clinic, which have health newsletters—tend to publish articles from only the most respected journals. However, you might have heard about an article some other way—for example, by going to Google Scholar or PubMed and typing in some keywords that bring up articles related to the topic.

The best journals only publish a fraction of the articles researchers submit to them—typically, 2 to 5 percent. Lower-quality journals will publish more articles to fill their pages, and the quality of the research might not be very good.

How do you judge whether a journal in which an article appeared is very reliable and selective about what they'll publish? You can look at the "IF."

## The "IF"

The impact factor, or the IF, is the medical research community's equivalent of the "It" factor in Hollywood. It corresponds to the number of times an article (or an average article) in a journal is cited in another article or publication. The best quality biomedical journals commonly have a high IF.

Every editor of a research journal wants their periodical to be the equivalent of the most-talked-about celebrity. How do editors get their new, not-yet-established journal to be the Hugh Jackman or Nicole Kidman of urology research journals? For one thing, they could publish a paper on the treatment of kidney stones that summarizes and references the latest research that happens to include the studies that have appeared in the journal previously. That article then gets online, and the next thing you know, the journal's studies have higher citation figures—in other words, a higher IF. On the journal's home page, the editor may include the IF, if it is high. You can do an internet search for "impact factor" and the name of the journal.

As a determined patient, you can ask a specialist what the highest-rated journals in their field are and check out the IF rating of any you come across that your specialist didn't mention. The title of the journal may sound impressive, but it may be the equivalent of a theater in a school somewhere in North Birdsfoot, Montana, compared to one on Broadway in New York City.

## Be Somewhat Skeptical about "Breakthrough" Studies

One advantage scientists and physicians have over many laypeople is that they know that true breakthroughs in science don't happen every day, so they have a healthy amount of skepticism. They look at the established science and all the research that has been done to date and consider it before getting too excited by a new study's remarkable results. Those roundup articles (or reviews) we mentioned before that cite all the research done so far are ones physicians know not to skip. You should consider reading them, too, in case they have more detail than what you'll find on the major websites and UptoDate.

Now that you know a little about quality studies and the journals that feature them, let's say you hear about a study on the news. There are a few things to be aware of before trying to track down the study itself.

When the researchers and physicians reporting results are the primary sources for the news release or article, they have a vested interested in presenting the results so as to make the research seem very important. After all, getting more grants for research and conducting studies is core to their job and their ability to get promotions and earn more money. In an ideal world, biomedical scientists would be completely objective about the research they plan to do—but they are like parents who are asked to be objective about their own children. It might be hard for researchers not to focus on the strengths of their study rather than any weaknesses. Reporters who cover the results are also supposed to be objective about the value of the study and its context, but their excitement over being able to report very important results could bias their reporting.

As an exercise, you might want to read several articles on the same study results that are about to be published in a medical journal. Note the differences in the reporting and ask yourself: Why did this journalist emphasize something different from what the other journalist emphasized? You might not be able to figure out the answer, but it will show you that reporters sometimes have a spin. That spin might not be helpful for you in your unique situation.

The truth is you won't often see a headline that says something like, "New Study Shows That Earlier Studies Are Correct: Immunosuppressant Drugs Work to Suppress Immunity," or "New High Blood Pressure Medication Performs Just as Well but Not Better Than Older Medications." Yet these types of studies add to our understanding of disease and treatment. When it comes to what seem to be breakthrough studies, it's up to the reader to be hopeful and optimistic but somewhat skeptical, too.

You should be especially concerned when the reporter relies on the author of a study as the *sole* source of information for a report. Often, the journalist is a generalist when it comes to health and might not pick up on important nuances to the study—and is relying on the study's author to point them out. The best news outlets make sure they have experts or key opinion leaders who were not involved in the study comment on the results and their significance.

In other words, newspaper reports are only a starting point for understanding health research. Sometimes they disclose important discoveries and new treatments. At other times, they raise false hopes. The first thing to do when you see or hear about some new information that seems like it may be of benefit to you is to reach out to your physician, who is most likely in a much better position to evaluate its validity and applicability to you. Your doctor might want to follow up with the study's investigators to learn more, or you might want to do it yourself. (The follow-up should be with the investigators themselves rather than the reporters or writers, who are only relaying the investigators' work). The investigators will be able to tell your doctor or you the stage their discovery or findings are at. For example, is the clinical trial an early one? Are the findings preliminary, or can they be applied to patients now? Additionally, the investigators may be able to direct you to the best way to access the treatment (perhaps through a specific medical center.)

## When Bad Research Slips Through

It could be that even after scrutiny by other researchers, a study may pass muster with a high-quality journal because no one spotted that the results were skewed due to an unseen factor—or recognized the limitations of the study. Research is imperfect.

Researchers try to anticipate anything that might affect their study's results and account for it, but sometimes, they overlook a factor that turns out to be important—even, sometimes, seemingly obvious ones, like temperature: How heart cells in a petri dish respond in the experiment done in a room that was 72 degrees Fahrenheit might not apply to how heart cells behave in a human body that has an internal temperature of 98.6 degrees. In a case like this, other researchers will try to duplicate the experiment and, if they do it in an environment with a temperature closer to 98 degrees, they might end up with different results.

Recently, thirty-one published papers by a cardiologist at Harvard Medical School, considered a KOL on stem cell research, were retracted by medical journals when it was found that he had falsified data that showed injecting stem cells into heart muscle can regenerate it. Another stem cell researcher, Kohei Yamamizu, associated with a center at Kyoto University in Japan that was directed by a Nobel Prize winner, was found guilty of falsifying images in a 2017 paper on stem cells. Sadly, some people are either so desperate to be right about their ideas or so desperate to be seen as cutting edge that they throw their ethics out the window.

Some studies have been retracted after it was found that researchers took financial kickbacks from drug companies whose medications were being studied. Not revealing funding sources that could sway a researcher to be biased violates professional ethics and the rules of medical journals. It doesn't happen often, but it isn't unheard of.

When a study doesn't seem to have been unduly influenced by the source of funding, or the researchers' strong desire to find a breakthrough blinding them to flaws in their research, a skeptic will still look at an original research study and see whether the math—the statistics—holds up. Recently, there has been a considerable amount of focus on statistics. For example, statisticians have suggested a raising of the bar when it comes to statistical analysis of scientific data. The hope is that this change would result in fewer questionable research studies getting published.

# How to Read a Journal Article on a Research Study

Reading research articles in peer-reviewed journals is generally considered the domain of experts, such as doctors and scientists, but you can conquer these yourself as a determined patient by studying them. If you're overwhelmed by the medical and academic language you have seen when clicking on a research study online, fear not: We're going to help you make sense of it. We'll also help you sort through which articles might apply to you and which won't.

For starters, if you don't have a serious medical condition, you can ignore basic studies. If you do, as we said earlier, you might want to contact the corresponding author of a basic research study that's been done on animals to see if you can access the treatment, which might go into a phase 1 clinical trial, because you're in dire circumstances and will likely get cleared for compassionate care.

When it comes to studies of people, you can always ask your doctor about a specific research study you came across. A specialist, in particular, may have read the study and have an opinion on it. Your doctor might be intrigued by the study you discovered and might agree to look at it and see if it yields information that can help you and other patients in your situation.

When you find an article that you think might be helpful to understand, you might just read the title and then the abstract or summary, which offers brief versions of each section, such as the objective, background, methodology, results, and conclusion (also known as a "discussion"). Some studies are set up so that the conclusion appears before the abstract. Your main interest is the conclusion and, secondarily, the various aspects of the study that are summarized in the abstract. The last thing you'll want to read will be the details of the study, which come after the abstract or summary.

Once you've read the latter, it might be best to talk with your doctor who can read the entire study and will have an easier time making sense of the very specific details. For one thing, your doctor will understand the statistical analysis—something few patients can do unless they've studied statistics. What you find in the abstract or summary may be enough to convince you that this study is worth discussing with your medical team—or that it isn't.

Let's look closer at reading a study's title and list of researchers and then look at the other parts of the article. Remember, you'll be looking at the abstract with its summaries of the aspects of the study first, and then, if you wish, you'll be looking at the details in the actual study.

## Title of the Article

Every research article has a title and often, but not always, it will tell you what the results of the study were. If you don't understand the language in the title, break down the language and look up each word. Let's look at the title of the mouse study mentioned earlier: "Combinatorial treatment of idiopathic pulmonary fibrosis using nanoparticles with prostaglandin E and siRNA(s)."

If you have idiopathic pulmonary fibrosis, you already know that it means your lungs (pulmonary) are developing fibrosis (scarring) for no known reason (idiopathic). "Combinatorial treatment" you can guess at or look up: It simply means combined treatment. Two treatments, nanoparticles with prostaglandin E and nanoparticles with siRNAs, were looked at in this study. If that wasn't clear to you, you could always read the article's abstract or summary to better understand what the study involved. In this case, the abstract says, "Inhalation delivery of prostaglandin E (PGE2) in combination with selected siRNA(s) was proposed for the efficient treatment of idiopathic pulmonary fibrosis (IPF)." That makes it very clear that the combination treatment studied was inhaling prostaglandin E and selected siRNAs.

Breaking down the title word by word, combined with reading the abstract/summary, should give you a clear sense of what was studied and what the results were. Note that the abstract/summary at the beginning of an article often has a section simply labeled "conclusion," which states the major finding of the study.

Let's say you come across a research study by using an internet search, but you don't know from the title of the study what it concluded and how its results apply to you. Or let's say you heard about the study from news reports and looked up the original research online. If you don't understand the language in the title or anywhere else in the study, you can consult the article for the general public that brought you to the study, if there is one— or look for such an article using keywords from the study's title to do your searching. With our pulmonary fibrosis article, you might want to look up "siRNA treatment pulmonary fibrosis," for example, and see if you can find an article in easy-to-understand language explaining what siRNA is and does. (Hint: it's a biological messenger that inhibits certain genes from expressing—siRNA is a hot topic in research showing promise for treating diseases that don't respond to many or perhaps even any medications.)

You can always break down the language of the title and in the abstract and look up each term that's used by consulting a dictionary (online, try www.Dictionary.com) or a health-care website such as WebMD. Generally speaking, if you do a search using Google, it will give some simple answers to questions such as: Which statin has the fewest side effects? and What can be done for fibromyalgia pain? If you read those, be sure to check the original source of the information. The website they're citing should end in .org, .gov, or .edu, which stand for "organization," "government," and "education." Many people are more familiar with sites that end in .com, which indicates a commercial site. These are less reliable for attaining medical information and definitions of terms.

You might also want to check YouTube, Khan Academy, or the website for an organization devoted to a particular condition, disease, or set of diseases, such as the American Cancer Society's website, to find a video with animation or visuals that can help you understand biological processes, procedures, and the way certain types of medications work. For example, the American Heart Association has videos on topics such as blood flow through the heart, angioplasty, and pacemakers, and illustrations and explanations of other topics, such as statin drugs. Khan Academy, a popular website for informational and instructional videos, has a series of videos on heart diseases and their treatments as well as videos and articles on autoimmune disorders and cancer. As you begin to better understand your condition or disease, you'll start to recognize terms and disease processes, making it easier for you to make sense of the language in research articles.

Let's look at another study:

"Radial-Artery or Saphenous-Vein Grafts in Coronary-Artery Bypass Surgery"

Coronary bypass surgery is a procedure for bypassing a blockage in an artery so that blood can continue to flow to the heart. The difference between a vein and an artery is that veins are smaller tubes with thinner walls and transport oxygen-poor blood back to the heart, which sends oxygen-rich blood back through the body via arteries. Arteries are bigger than veins and have thicker, more flexible walls.

The title of the article still might confuse you at this point, but you can look up "radial artery" (it's an artery in the forearm) and "saphenous vein" (it's a vein in the leg). The article is about grafting one or the other onto the clogged artery so there's a new avenue for blood to flow to the heart.

## List of the Study's Researchers

After the study's title comes the list of the researchers involved in the study. As explained earlier in the chapter, the research team includes the researcher who designed and set up the study as well as the lead author of the study, and those could be the same person. The rest of the team is listed as well. The first and last names in the research team list tend to be the important names because those individuals headed up the team in some way. As a general convention in biomedical publications, the first author is the one who did most of the experimental work and the last (or senior) author is the person in whose laboratory the project was conceived and the work was done. As noted earlier, the researcher listed as the "corresponding author" is the person you should contact if you have any questions about the study. His or her contact information should be listed, sometimes in a section called "correspondence." If you want to speak to the key opinion leader involved in the study, speak first to the corresponding author.

## Abstract or Summary of the Article

Now let's look at the parts of an actual study, which are summed up in shorter sections in the abstract or summary. Note that the conclusion, a short statement, might appear before the abstract or at the end of it. Either way, read the conclusion after you've made sense of the study's title. Then, read the abstract. If the conclusion is, in essence, "this treatment is no better than earlier treatments," there's no point in reading on. If the conclusion is positive and you want to read more, you could read the entire study from beginning to end, but you might not be able to make sense of all the details. That's okay—your doctor can help you with any questions, assuming your doctor is willing to work with you as a determined patient and discuss research that might apply to you.

The parts of the abstract or summary are generally the introduction/background, methods, results, and, as mentioned, the conclusion. (Again, each of these is substantially expanded upon in the body of the report.) Let's look a little more closely at each of these summarizing pieces:

*Introduction/Background.* The abstract is the condensed version of the article. It offers an introduction to the justification for and purpose of the study (for example, the need for stopping the progression of pulmonary fibrosis or for doing surgery to bypass blocked veins) and gives some background information about what's already known. Then, the authors identify critical gaps in the field. The purpose or objective of the study is usually to fill in one of the gaps. A valuable part of the introduction is any reference to landmark articles and review articles on the general topic. These might be worth reading if you need additional background information on the topic to understand the article.

*Methodology/Methods (in the Abstract and the Study).* The introduction in the abstract is generally followed by a short methods section, also known as a methodology section, which spells out how the study was done. Among other things, it will tell you the specific experimental techniques that were used. For example, maybe it's an observational study that analyzed patient outcomes and records rather than types of experiments performed in a laboratory. Maybe it's a review of studies. The article on vein vs. artery bypasses lists in its methodology that it is a review of six studies and "mixed-effects Cox regression models were used to estimate the treatment effect on the outcomes." That's a common methodology for analyzing survival statistics in a group of people being studied.

To a person knowledgeable in the field, the methods section is extremely important since it may highlight the strengths and weaknesses of the study. You might learn in this section that the study you're reading followed a certain group of patients from the time they first began taking a medication until thirty days after they stopped. Another study might have looked at a similar group of patients who had been taking a medication for five years or more. Some studies, including many nutritional studies, are based on patient reporting—for example, reporting of the foods they have consumed. In a case like this, testing for certain nutrients in the blood before, during, and after the study may or may not have been done. Researchers will often explain why they made certain choices about the methodology.

The methodology section is probably the most difficult section for someone not trained in the field or in statistics to analyze or evaluate, so it's something you might want to discuss with a doctor rather than try to figure it out yourself.

***Results (within the Abstract or the Study).*** The results section generally comes after the methods section within the abstract, but in the paper itself, the two sections may be combined. The results section in the study itself presents data from the study, outcomes, and—typically—graphs and tables. The authors of the research article will walk the reader through the logic for doing each of the experiments if more than one is involved. If it is a clinical study, it will generally start with the characteristics of the patient population studied, such as the average ages and range of ages of the subjects, their weights and heights, ethnicities, comorbidities, etc. For example, in the vein vs. artery bypass study we have been looking at, the results section of the abstract reads as follows:

A total of 1,036 patients were included in the analysis (534 patients with radial-artery grafts and 502 patients with saphenous-vein grafts). After a mean ($\pm$SD) follow-up time of 60$\pm$30 months, the incidence of adverse cardiac events was significantly lower in association with radial-artery grafts than with saphenous-vein grafts (hazard ratio, 0.67; 95% confidence interval [CI], 0.49 to 0.90; P=0.01). At follow-up angiography (mean follow-up, 50$\pm$30 months), the use of radial-artery grafts was also associated with a significantly lower risk of occlusion (hazard ratio, 0.44; 95% CI, 0.28 to 0.70; P<0.001). As compared with the use of saphenous-vein grafts, the use of radial-artery grafts was associated with a nominally lower incidence of myocardial infarction (hazard ratio, 0.72; 95% CI, 0.53 to 0.99; P=0.04) and a lower incidence of repeat revascularization (hazard ratio, 0.50; 95% CI, 0.40 to 0.63; P<0.001) but not a lower incidence of death from any cause (hazard ratio, 0.90; 95% CI, 0.59 to 1.41; P=0.68).

If you don't understand the statistics here (and you probably won't), you can see that the 534 patients who had radial-artery grafts had fewer cardiac events, a lower risk of occlusion (blockage), and a lower incidence of needing another bypass surgery—even if they died at the same rate the 502 patients who had saphenous-vein grafts did.

So does that mean you should seek a radial-artery graft rather than a saphenous-vein graft? Take a look at the conclusion or discussion next, as it summarizes the study's results and addresses their relevance or importance.

***Conclusion or Discussion (within the Abstract).*** The final section of the abstract/summary or full report is called either the discussion or the conclusion. This might be the most valuable (and most efficient) place to start in evaluating and understanding the article's potential relevance to you. In the case of our example, the conclusion in the abstract/summary states simply:

As compared with the use of saphenous-vein grafts, the use of radial-artery grafts for CABG resulted in a lower rate of adverse cardiac events and a higher rate of patency at 5 years of follow-up.

That might sound more like a results section than a conclusion section, but often, the conclusion will be more definitive, reporting what treatments and interventions the data support.

**Funding (within the Abstract or the Study).** There's another section of a research article you should know about and that is the one that identifies how the study was funded. Checking the funding source for the research, which is either within the abstract or at the end of the study, can help you spot potential biases that may have affected the outcomes. Ideally, you want to see that the research was funded by branches of the federal government (for example, the National Institutes of Health) or organizations that have no commercial interest in the outcome (findings) of the study, such as the Bill and Melinda Gates Foundation, the Rockefeller Foundation, or the American College of Cardiology.

After reading the sections of the abstract, consider looking at the details of the study. Is there more you want to know? Or would it be best to talk with your doctor about the details? In any case, after reading the research article, if you ask your doctor about the research and the differences between you and those who participated, you will have a richer conversation than if you simply asked, "My friend had a vein taken from his leg when he had bypass surgery, so why are you suggesting taking an artery from my arm instead?" Here's the bottom line: Read the abstract, and if you think that the results or conclusion are relevant to your situation, talk to your doctor about the quality of the study and its applicability to you—and consider reading the details in the rest of the study.

## What Now?

We hope this chapter has helped you better understand research studies and how to make sense of them so that with the help your doctor, you can make more informed choices about treatments. Learning about your disease or condition will not happen overnight, but wherever you are in your understanding of your health issues and what can be done to treat them, always keep in mind that there is no such thing as a "dumb question" when it comes to your health.

---

## Notes on Reading Journal Articles on Research

- Basic studies on cells and animals and studies done on people—whether they are clinical trials or observational studies—can yield valuable information about human health and how to treat diseases and conditions. Studies of studies can help us make sense of seemingly contradictory results of different studies.

- Longitudinal studies follow participants for a long time, are expensive to run, and give us some of the very best information about diseases and treatments.

- When deciding whether it's worth looking closely at a research study, be sure it's in a respected, peer-reviewed journal with a high IF (impact factor) and that the funding source isn't questionable.

- Statistics, specific methodologies considered legitimate by the research community, and peer review help a study to be one of the rare 2 to 5 percent of studies submitted to prestigious, reliable medical journals that are accepted. Even so, sometimes research is faked or not reproducible and therefore unreliable. Remember: Newer isn't always better.

- Medications are tested in clinical trials that have phases, but medical devices are studied using observation, statistics, and well-accepted methodologies that help researchers determine the benefits and drawbacks of the device.

- A video of a procedure or test or how a medical device or medication works in the body can be helpful. Look for them at the website for a major organization dedicated to your disease or a video site that offers tutorials (check who created the video to make sure it's from a reliable source).

- The abstract of a study offers short versions of the sections within the actual study. It's important to see what the research was looking at, how the study was conducted, and what the results and conclusion were. Whatever you don't understand, you can look up using the internet and discuss with your doctor.

- Don't rely entirely on an article for the general public that summarizes the results of a research study. Check the original study and discuss it with your doctor if it feels appropriate to do so.

## A Last Word

We hope that as a determined patient, you are feeling encouraged to believe you have the power to get better health outcomes than you've been getting to date—and better access to quality care than you've had in the past. There will probably be times when you're confused by what you discover in your research or hear from your doctor. You may feel intimidated asking questions or overwhelmed by the task of self-advocating, particularly when a doctor doesn't seem to want to partner with you so much as have you see them as the expert who shouldn't be questioned. Simply saying, "I'm determined to know as much as I can and do as much as I can to get the best health outcome possible," can remind your doctor that you want to have a partnership that involves respect for each other, honesty, and a shared goal: better health for you. As doctors, we love to see our patients get better and know that we made a significant difference in improving their lives. It's why we got into medicine in the first place.

So, know where your power lies—in being determined to take charge of your health, partner effectively with your doctor, and let nothing stand in your way as you work to achieve optimal health. You've got this!

# ENDNOTES

## Chapter 2: Determined to Partner with Professionals

1. Medical fraud case in New York. CBS New York, "Cardiologist Sentenced to 6 ½ Years for $19 Million Billing Fraud," New York CBS Local, November 20, 2013. http://newyork.cbslocal.com/2013/11/20/cardiologist-sentenced-to-78-months-for-19-million-billing-fraud/

2. Medical fraud news from the U.S. Department of Justice. https://www.justice.gov/criminal-fraud/news-and-noteworthy

3. Doctors' reputations not following them from state to state. Matt Wynn, "There's a Tool to Help States Find Problem Doctors. Why Do So Few Use It?" *Milwaukee Journal Sentinel/MedPage Today*, March 7, 2018. https://www.jsonline.com/story/news/investigations/2018/03/07/theres-tool-help-states-find-problem-doctors-why-do-so-few-use/400723002/

## Chapter 4: Determined to Follow Through on Your Treatment

1. East Coast insurer flies patients to Mexico for knee surgery. Phil Galewitz, "A Mexican Hospital, an American

Surgeon, and a $5000 Check (Yes, a Check)," *New York Times,* Business section, August 9, 2019. https://www.nytimes.com/2019/08/09/business/medical-tourism-mexico.html?fbclid=IwAR0tAFDy2k_EiCeY3VyyLGal3GH-Wu7mZ8dEHdzHKtNuZICgPOEJKB-N01mw

2. Josef Woodman and Jeremy Abbate, *Patients Beyond Borders: Everybody's Guide to Affordable, World-Class Medical Travel.* (Chapel Hill, NC: Healthy Travel Media, third edition, 2015).

## Chapter 5: Determined to Turn Over Every Stone

1. Hormone replacement therapy (HRT) trial halted. JoAnn Manson et al., "Menopausal Hormone Therapy and Health Outcomes During the Intervention and Extended Poststopping Phases of the Women's Health Initiative Randomized Trials," *Journal of the American Medical Association* 310(13):1353–1358, October 2, 2013. https://jamanetwork.com/journals/jama/fullarticle/1745676

2. Reproducibility is a "significant crisis." Monya Baker, "1500 Scientists Lift the Lid on Reproducibility," *Nature* 533(7604), May 25, 2016. https://www.nature.com/news/1-500-scientists-lift-the-lid-on-reproducibility-1.19970

## Chapter 6: Determined to Understand

1. Pulmonary fibrosis mouse study. O.B. Garbuzneko et al., "Combinatorial treatment of idiopathic pulmonary fibrosis using nanoparticles with prostaglandin E and siRNA(s)," *Nanomedicine* 13(6):1983–1992, August 2017. https://pubmed.ncbi.nlm.nih.gov/28434932/

2. Artery and vein study. M. Gardino et al., "Radial-Artery or Saphenous-Vein Grafts in Coronary-Artery Bypass Surgery,"

*New England Journal of Medicine* 378(22):2069–2077, May 31, 2018. http://ncbi.nlm.nih.gov/pubmed/29708851

3. Thirty-one stem cell research papers by researcher at Harvard Medical School retracted. Gina Kolata, "Harvard Calls for Retraction of Dozens of Studies by Noted Cardiac Researcher," *New York Times*, Health section, October 15, 2018. https://www.nytimes.com/2018/10/15/health/piero-anversa-fraud-retractions.html

4. Stem cell research paper retracted due to falsified images. "Researcher at Japan Stem Cell Institute Falsified Nearly All Images in 2017 Paper," Bioethics.com, January 24, 2018. https://bioethics.com/archives/41783

# RESOURCES

If you'd like to learn more about your diagnosis, or if you're not sure it's the correct one, you might want to check WebMD and www.MedicineNet.com and their related sites. You might also want to check an official site dedicated to the understanding and treatment of your disease or the bodily system it affects, such as the Pulmonary Fibrosis Foundation website or the American Heart Association website, for example.

The National Cancer Institute's list of NCI-Designated Cancer Centers can be found at https://www.cancer.gov/research/infrastructure/cancer-centers

To discover the latest information about treatments for medical conditions, go to www.UptoDate.com. You can access the same information about your condition that your doctor is reading. It costs about $20 for a seven-day trial subscription, which you can cancel after doing your research.

*U.S. News & World Report's* annual hospital rankings can be found on their website at https://health.usnews.com/best-hospitals/rankings

You can comparison shop for nonemergency testing through these sites:

http://www.NewChoiceHealth.com

http://Health.Costhelper.com

http://www.ClearHealthCosts.com

You can find the website for your state's medical board through an internet search and use it to double-check that a physician genuinely is board certified. You can also look up doctors on the website of the American Board of Internal Medicine (ABIM), the American Board of Medical Specialties (ABMS), and other boards, such as the American Board of Family Medicine (ABFM), to assure yourself that they are currently board certified. You can also visit the FBI's website at https://www.fbi.gov/scams-and-safety/common-scams-and-crimes/health-care-fraud to see their press releases on health-care frauds they've discovered.

If you're interested in medical tourism, you might want to look at the book *Patients Beyond Borders: Everybody's Guide to Affordable, World-Class Medical Travel* by Josef Woodman and Jeremy Abbate, third edition (Chapel Hill, NYC: Healthy Travel Media, 2015).

You can find research studies through searches of Google Scholar (https://scholar.google.com/) or PubMed (https://www.ncbi.nlm.nih.gov/pubmed/). Note that often, the abstract is available for free but you have to pay to access an individual article. A medical library or university library might allow you to use their subscription to access the complete article for the sake of researching your medical condition, if you ask them.

You can check on the safety and effectiveness of medical devices at

https://www.fda.gov/medical-devices/medical-device-safety.

You can look up clinical trials that are starting up or underway at www.clinicaltrials.gov.

You can do an internet search for the impact factor (IF) of a journal or look it up at www.researchgate.net/directory/publications.

Made in the USA
Monee, IL
19 February 2022